WOMEN AND DISABILITY

WOMEN AND WORLD DEVELOPMENT SERIES

This series has been developed by the JUNIC Group on Women and Development and makes available the most recent information, debate and action being taken on world development issues, and the impact on women. Each volume is fully illustrated and attractively presented. Each outlines its particular subject, as well as including an introduction to resources and guidance on how to use the books in workshops and seminars. The aim of each title is to bring women's concerns more directly and effectively into the development process, and to achieve an improvement in women's status in our rapidly changing world.

The Group was established in 1980 to organise the production and distribution of joint UN/NGO development education materials. It was the first time that United Nations agencies and non-governmental organisations had collaborated in this way, and the Group remains a unique example of cooperation between international and non-governmental institutions. Membership of the Programme Group is open to all interested organisations.

SERIES TITLES – in order of scheduled publication

- **WOMEN AND THE WORLD ECONOMIC CRISIS**
  PREPARED BY JEANNE VICKERS

- **WOMEN AND DISABILITY**
  PREPARED BY ESTHER R. BOYLAN

- **WOMEN AND HEALTH**
  PREPARED BY PATRICIA SMYKE

- **REFUGEE WOMEN**
  PREPARED BY SUSAN FORBES MARTIN

- **WOMEN AND LITERACY**
  PREPARED BY MARCELA BALLARA

- **WOMEN AND THE ENVIRONMENT**
  PREPARED BY ANNABEL RODDA

- **WOMEN AT WORK**

- **WOMEN AND THE FAMILY**

For full details, as well as order forms, please write to:
ZED BOOKS LTD, 57 CALEDONIAN ROAD, LONDON N1 9BU, U.K.

WOMEN AND DISABILITY

PREPARED BY ESTHER BOYLAN

Zed Books Ltd · London & New Jersey

Women and Disability was first published by Zed Books Ltd,
57 Caledonian Road, London N1 9BU, United Kingdom and 165 First Avenue,
Atlantic Highlands, New Jersey 07716, United States of America, in 1991.

Copyright © United Nations Non-Governmental Liaison Service, 1991

Cover and book design by Lee Robinson
Cover photo: Anita Andersson
Typeset by Goodfellow & Egan, Cambridge
Printed and bound in the United Kingdom at The Bath Press, Avon

British Library Cataloguing in Publication Data

A catalogue record for this book is available from the British Library
ISBN 0 86232 986 8 hb
ISBN 0 86232 987 6 pb

Library of Congress Cataloging-in-Publication Data

Women and disability / prepared by Esther Boylan.
p. cm. — (Women and world development series)
Includes bibliographical references and index.
ISBN 0 86232 986 8 (cloth). — ISBN 0 86232 987 6 (paper)
1. Handicapped women—Social conditions.   2. Handicapped women—Developing
countries—Social conditions.   3. Rural women—Developing countries—Social
conditions.   4. Handicapped women—Rehabilitation.   I. Boylan, Esther.   II.
Series.
HV1569.3.W65W66   1991
362.4"082—dc20

91–12443
CIP

11-23-93

CONTENTS

ACKNOWLEDGEMENTS

The Joint UN/NGO Group on Women and Development wishes to acknowledge and thank the following organisations for their participation in the preparation of this book:

CO-ORDINATION OF THE UPDATE OF THIS BOOK

- International Labour Organisation (ILO), Vocational Rehabilitation Branch

THIS BOOK WAS MADE POSSIBLE BY FINANCIAL CONTRIBUTIONS FROM:

- United Nations Centre for Social Development and Humanitarian Affairs (CSDHA)
  - Division for the Advancement of Women
  - Disabled Persons' Unit
  - Voluntary Fund for United Nations Decade of Disabled Persons
- Middle East Committee for the Welfare of the Blind, Regional Bureau
- Norway – Norges Rode Kors, ET NYTT LIV (Norwegian Red Cross, A New Life)
- Rehabilitation International

The content of this book has been approved by the Joint UN/NGO Group on Women and Development, which wishes to thank all those United Nations specialised agencies, non-governmental organisations and individuals who generously contributed articles and information towards the preparation of this book. References and credits are to be found wherever these were used. The following organisations have made a special contribution through their participation in the editorial panel formed for this publication:

- Disabled Peoples' International
- IMPACT (a combined initiative of the United nations Development Programme, UNDP, WHO and UNICEF)
- Inter-African Committee on Traditional Practices
- International Council of Jewish Women
- League of Red Cross and Red Crescent Societies
- Lutheran World Federation
- Rehabilitation International
- United Nations Children's Fund (UNICEF)
- CSDHA
  - Division for the Advancement of Women
  - Disabled Persons' Unit
- World Council of Churches
- World Health Organisation (WHO)

Overall coordination and management of the Joint UN/NGO Group on Women and Development is provided by the UN Non-Governmental Liaison Service (NGLS), an inter--agency unit which fosters dialogue and cooperation between the UN system and the NGO community on development policy and North-South relations.

Explanatory note

WOMEN AND DISABILITY was first prepared in 1981, in the form of a kit, as a contribution to the International Year of Disabled Persons. The United Nations recently decided to update it because of the importance of the subject and because of the interest that it has aroused.

Contributions for the present document, now published as a book, were received from a number of specialised agencies of the United Nations, non-governmental organisations, professionals and disabled women themselves. While the international response was gratifying in its volume, its coverage was not as even as had been hoped. More articles were received about disabled women living in cities of industrial countries than about those in rural areas of the developing world. As a result, the picture that this book provides about the situation and the problems of women with disabilities does not tell the full story. It does, however, point out where we need to know more.

The book has been written with a very broad readership in mind. It is hoped that it will prove useful not only to international, governmental and non-governmental organisations but also to those working towards social development, to those in favour of the advancement of women in general, and of disabled women in particular. It is aimed, as well, at rehabilitation professionals and workers, and at disabled women and men and their families and their communities.

The main purpose of this book is to provide information about the special problems women with disabilities face in simply surviving and in trying to find their proper place within their families and in the cities, towns and villages where they live. Some of the subjects discussed may be controversial, which means that, as with everything, there is more than one way to see the real picture. For the real picture may appear different to different people depending upon their particular role, their attitudes and the power they may have to make things happen.

Articles, or portions of articles, that are reproduced in this book are listed in italics in the table of contents. *Women and Disability* will appear in the following language versions: English, French, Spanish and Arabic. It is also intended to produce a version for persons with visual handicaps.

ESTHER BOYLAN

What do 'DISABILITY' and 'HANDICAP' mean?

There is a difference between disability and handicap.

■ Disabled persons are not handicapped in all circumstances or in everything they do. Disability should, in no way, be seen as inability.

■ Disability may be permanent. When someone loses a leg in an accident, this disabling condition will remain throughout the person's lifetime. It may be a handicap in, for example, walking, riding a bicycle or working as a waitress, but not while playing card games, cooking a meal or working as a computer operator.

■ Concentrating on her ability – and not on what she cannot do – should be the principal concern of every disabled woman and of those agencies and individuals interested in her welfare.

FOREWORD
BY MARY
CHINERY-HESSE*

EQUALITY OF OPPORTUNITY and treatment for women has yet to be achieved in most societies. A woman with a physical or mental disability faces a double handicap.

This updated book on women and disability, however, gives us reason for optimism. It succinctly identifies the complex problems of disability among women, and paves the way for action and for working out solutions.

Why focus on the impact of disability on women when it certainly is not a problem unique to women? Whatever statistics we have on the issue – and these are scant – show that being female and having a disability, whether serious or not, is usually enough to put the individual in a very disadvantaged situation. Although some progress has been made in improving the status of women in general, disabled women have remained a largely ignored group. This has often led to unnecessary and undue hardships, and even to tragedy.

There is a great responsibility upon us all, whether in international, national or local service, to influence others and to help disabled women acquire a sense of self worth and achieve a sense of dignity. If the key message in this book comes across – the realisation that, regardless of our limitations, we are all members of the human race to which we can, in our own way, make a contribution given the appropriate skills and support; that the stigma of dependency and being a burden on society need not be attached to the disabled; that society as a whole stands to gain by adopting positive approaches to disability – then the efforts in preparing this document will have been worthwhile.

The confidence that this book will inspire in disabled women will ultimately be translated, I feel certain, into very concrete achievements in the workplace and in all aspects of daily life. And perhaps equally important, it will foster an enlightened attitude among the able-bodied as to the important role people with disabilities can play in a nation's economy and in society.

This book also seeks to make a contribution to increased international awareness. It presents the situation of disabled women eloquently through their own words and experiences which, in their unique way, can serve as inspiration for all.

---

* Deputy Director-General, International Labour Office

INTRODUCTION –
FROM AWARENESS
TO ACTION

A CHANCE ENCOUNTER on a Paris street, when a young actor stopped to comfort a tearful mother with a handicapped child, sparked a concern for severely handicapped persons and their parents that inspired the young man to wage a successful campaign on their behalf. His efforts brought about a recent change in French law that commits the government to providing proper homes for individuals who are profoundly handicapped.[1] Just one person can make a difference.

Although this book, which is the updated version of the JUNIC/NGO *Women and Disability* kit, is designed as a source of information and guidelines for action to improve the quality of life of women with disabilities, it could itself also provide a 'casual encounter'.

By adopting a less structured format and a more general approach, the updated book may serve as both a reminder and an eye-opener to a wider audience both within and beyond the disabled world. It may also inspire awareness of, it not action by, individuals and groups who previously knew nothing of the plight of women with disability. It may show women who are themselves disabled the possibilities and rewards that personal involvement in their own destiny can bring.

This updated book may also be seen as an opportunity to take stock following the International Year of Disabled Persons (1981), the United Nations Decade of Women (1976–85) and now the United Nations Decade of Disabled Persons (1983–92) as it moves towards its conclusion.

There is a disturbing similarity between two statements made just prior to the beginning of the Decade of Women and at its conclusion, the first by Rehabilitation International to the United Nations in June 1975, the second by the World Conference to Review the Achievements of the Decade, held in Nairobi in July 1985:

Both of the statements emphasise the special predicament of women who are disabled in access to the lives of their societies. Both statements refer to the disproportionate burden of coping with disability which is shouldered by women in any society. There really is no significant difference in concept between these two position statements. The fact that one was made at the beginning of the United Nations Decade of Women and the other was expressed at the conclusion of the Decade, at a point near to the mid-point of the Decade of Disabled Persons, is not at all apparent from the issues to which they refer.

Neither in concept, nor in goals, nor in the difficult reality which continues to be faced by disabled women throughout the world has there been any serious change from the beginning to the end of the Decade of Women.[2]

At the Nairobi Conference there was not a single woman with disability in any national delegation except that from Australia. Furthermore, when nearly 100 women with disability, not delegates, assembled daily for a workshop in conjunction with the conference, they assembled outdoors because the facilities provided were 'inaccessible' ... fortunately the conference was not held in the winter in a cold climate.

SELF-HELP, A RECURRING THEME □
The workshop itself was yet another

indication that disabled women are increasingly searching for a common voice and are claiming their rights as members of the human race. Self-help is a theme that more and more frequently runs through the programmes, projects, recommendations and conclusions reached by organisations and agencies concerned with women and disability.

The United Nations Decade of Disabled Persons is intended as a time-frame for implementing the World Programme of Action concerning Disabled Persons, which was a major outcome of the International Year of Disabled Persons. But the World Programme of Action itself was found wanting by a meeting of experts, composed mostly of persons with disability, which was held in Stockholm in August 1987 to evaluate the implementation of the programme. The meeting concluded that the programme failed to place adequate emphasis on the needs of women who are disabled and that particular attention should be given to the improvement of their situation.

Despite shortcomings in some areas, more and more sustained and co-ordinated efforts are being made by governmental, inter-governmental and non-governmental organisations (NGOs) to help women with disabilities, bringing rays of hope into their shadowy world. Such women are becoming a preoccupation of such NGOs as Rehabilitation International (RI) which is working to bring about a change in the situation confronting disabled women. The world congresses, organised every four years through its network of 120 member organisations in 80 countries to focus public attention on issues related to disability prevention and rehabilitation, include specific topics on women and disability.

Some other NGOs have special committees and memberships that consist mostly of women with disability. Disabled Peoples' International (DPI), for example, has a Standing Committee on Affairs of Women with Disability and convenes special training seminars and workshops. The World Blind Union (WBU) Committee on the Status of Blind Women has sponsored training seminars for them. The World Association of Girl Scouts and Girl Guides has several projects concerned with disabled girls. Other NGOs, including the International Federation of Ageing and the International Federation of Multiple Sclerosis Societies, also undertake special studies concerned with disabled women.

NEW AREAS OF INTEREST □ As well as dealing with familiar concerns such as prevention, education and rehabilitation with reference to women and disability, this updated book brings other areas of interest into the spotlight with new sections on subjects such as caregivers ('...in the Shadow of Disability', chapter 5), ageing women and disability ('Growing Older: a Time to Endure... or Enjoy?', chapter 6), and some of the ways in which women who are disabled are breaking out of the cocoon of disability ('New Horizons: Taking Control', chapter 7).

Helping women with disabilities to achieve full participation and equality depends upon positive and constructive attitudes. Without these, even the most sophisticated technologies may be ineffective. It is to foster the combined efforts that are needed to bring about a change in attitudes that this book has been prepared.

1 Barry James, 'One man's fight for the handicapped', *International Herald Tribune*, 24 February 1989.
2 'Women and disability', Susan R. Hammerman, Secretary-General, Rehabilitation International to the Rehabilitation International Conference on Women with Disabilities, New York, February 1986.

THE STIGMA OF DISABILITY

Many women are handicapped – discriminated against merely because they are women. Having a disability compounds this prejudice, particularly for women in developing countries where the majority of the millions of disabled women can be found. For them, disability diminishes sharply their often inferior role, even in their own households. The stigma of disability, with its myths and fears, increases their social isolation. When no rehabilitation facilities are available, they become immobile and housebound, and their isolation is complete.

To say that women with disability suffer not only the usual discrimination against females but also are further discriminated against because of their disability is, perhaps, to state the obvious. Nevertheless, this double prejudice is the root cause of the inferior status of women with disabilities, making them the world's most disadvantaged group. It is the cause of hostility and negative attitudes that are often more debilitating for disabled women than the disability itself.

DISABILITY AND ITS CHALLENGES □

No one is immune from becoming disabled and, in a world on the threshold of a new century, the chief causes of disability are still very much with us, especially malnutrition, which has disabled millions of women in developing countries.

Life is less bleak for women with disability in industrialised countries, where recent biomedical and technological developments offer remarkable new opportunities. Here, there is improved access to education and skills, and computer-based technologies that compensate for disabilities of various kinds. Infants born at high risk have a better chance of surviving difficult births without disabling trauma through better and comprehensive natal and medical care.

> Her inferior status in society is often more debilitating for a disabled woman than the disability itself.

There has also been an extraordinary growth in the participation of people who are themselves disabled in determining the best approaches and programmes to meet their needs and the needs of their families. This has sparked among disabled people an increasing sense of self-worth, self-respect and dignity, qualities that are at the core of the disabled woman's capacity to improve her own life.

Moreover, new concepts for activating all members of the community have been developed which have the potential to revolutionise the quality of life of people with disabilities through community-based rehabilitation measures. Studies of the situations of disabled people, particularly women and young children, in developing countries show that they enjoy practically none of these improvements.

Too much work, too little food □

According to findings by the International Labour Organisation (ILO), in general women in rural areas of developing countries work from twelve to sixteen hours a day, doing the bulk of agricultural work and the marketing and processing of produce, after which they remain exclusively responsible for all domestic chores and the care of children and dependants.

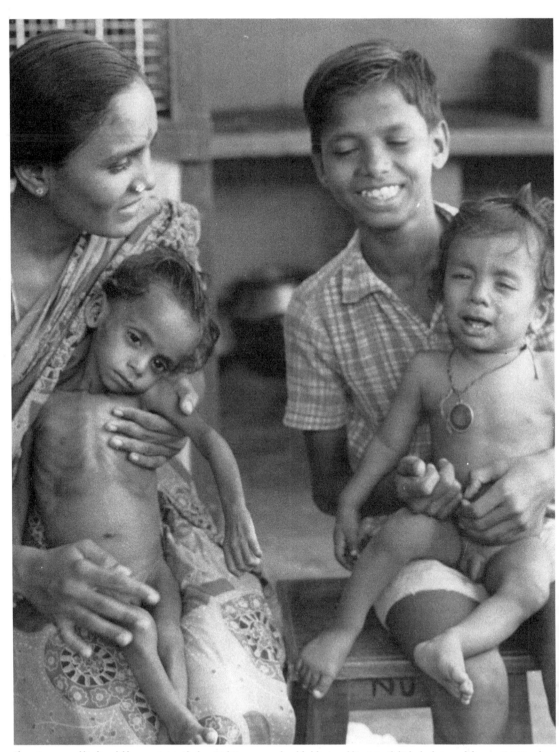

These two-year-old Indian children are twins. The boy (right) was nursed and fed first, and his sister (left) had what was left over. Nutritional rehabilitation centre at C.S.I. Campbell Hospital, Jammalamadugu, southern India.

It is not surprising, then, that millions of these women are: ... permanently in poor health, not from specific illness, but from general maternal depletion caused by too much work and too little food combined with too many pregnancies too close together. From girlhood to womanhood, females in many societies are fed last and least... Under these conditions, major causes of impairment and disability among children – infectious diseases, malnutrition of pregnant mother and child, injuries before or at birth, accidents and other sources of trauma – are the least controlled.[1]

In developing countries, a woman's status is considered to be subjugated and dependent.

When she becomes disabled she loses her status altogether as there are often no facilities provided to rehabilitate her in her role. Thus she becomes totally isolated, immobile and confined to the house. It is much more difficult for her than it is for a male with disability to participate in public activities or meetings, unless special efforts are made to help her do so

For her, there is no disability allowance, no environmental adjustment, practically no access to education or training and therefore to employment, and no opportunity to become involved in self-help movements.

As far as the marriage problem is concerned, the situation of disabled women in developing countries is much more difficult, as marriages are mostly arranged. Stereotyped concepts, prejudices and negative attitudes about disability are so deeply rooted that they greatly influence these arrangements.[2]

It may be assumed that the number of disabled people living in the rural areas of this [Asian] region are in the same proportion as in the general population, 65 to 80 per cent. However, the facilities and services available for them exist in reverse proportion, 90 per cent in the urban areas and hardly 10 per cent in rural areas. This, combined with the fact that the environment barriers – both structural and attitudinal – traditional patterns and deep-rooted prejudices against disability are far more intense in the rural areas and more difficult to change, makes the situation of disabled people in rural areas far worse than those in urban areas.[3]

Families in rural areas do not send even able-bodied girls to school once they attain puberty. Education and training are seen as investment in breadwinners. Man is seen as a breadwinner and the woman's role is seen as wife and mother.[4]

Even within the sisterhood of women with disabilities, there are those whose handicaps provoke even further discrimination, particularly the mentally retarded and the blind.

Devalued as she is for being a woman, subject to deep prejudice due to her disability, and dismissed for the unaccepted manner in which she may articulate her needs and desires, the woman who has a mental handicap is at enormous risk of being invisible and without a voice. Not surprisingly, this has profound consequences in terms of both the quality of life experienced by most women with intellectual impairments and the options which are open to them.

It is estimated that between 80 and 90 per cent of all persons labelled as mentally handicapped are unemployed. For most, who are forced to live on social assistance, chronic poverty is the norm. Many women continue to work in segregated settings (sheltered workshops) where they are paid to carry out routine tasks for well below the minimum wage.[5]

Attitudes and ignorance are particularly virulent where blind women are concerned – no one would readily consider marrying off a blind girl or asking for her hand in marriage. Objects of false pity and

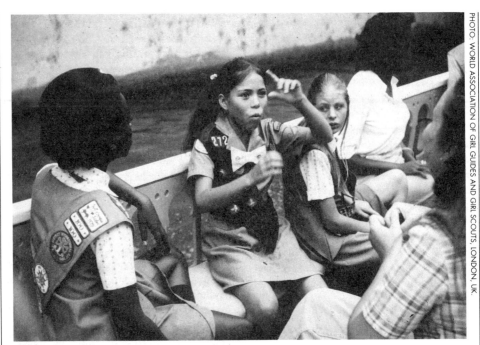

PHOTO: WORLD ASSOCIATION OF GIRL GUIDES AND GIRL SCOUTS, LONDON, UK.

Girl Scouts from the USA proving that disability is not a barrier.

mindless charity, blind women are often relegated to the lowest status in the community – they are isolated from society and confined to a corner of the house and live in obscurity, silent misery and total social and economic dependency.

By actively responding to the plight of their disabled peers, including those who are mentally and visually handicapped, Girl Guides and Girl Scouts throughout the world are setting a shining example of compassion and constructive help that puts to shame the passive indifference too often found in the adult world. Girl Guide and Girl Scout groups in Nigeria, Bangladesh and the Republic of Korea are active in projects that include a vocational training centre for disabled girls, a school for mentally retarded children and fundraising for a school for blind children. An important feature of the Girl Guide/Girl Scout movement is the integration of disabled girls as members or, in

some cases, the formation of special units for them.

The lowest in the hierarchy of women with disabilities – and the most invisible – are certainly the disabled women among the uprooted populations who have fled violence in their own countries and live in refugee camps, often under rigorous conditions, making them particularly vulnerable to mental and psychosomatic problems.

No one knows how many of the world's 15 million refugees suffer physical or mental disability. Relatively little research has been undertaken to assess their needs and individual capacities. The disabled refugees are 'victims among the victims' of conflicts and wars in Afghanistan, Angola, Ethiopia, Kampuchea, Mozambique, Somalia, Sri Lanka and Sudan.

The massive problems faced by international and national organisations in their efforts to help the ever-growing numbers of refugees tend to eclipse the particular problems of disabled people among them. Yet an increasing number of projects is being launched to provide them with medical care and physical aids. Though relatively few non-governmental organisations specialise in assistance to disabled refugees, two are particularly active in this field: Handicap International, a French agency, and Okenden Venture, based in the United Kingdom (UK).

A blueprint for action □ Current projections suggest that the world's population will increase by 90 million each year until the year 2000, with all but 6 million of each year's increase occurring in the Third World.

The implications of this forecast for already overpopulated developing countries are catastrophic. A call to arms was sounded at the international level in May 1989, in the annual report of the United Nations Fund for Population Activities. The report urged that investment in women be made to 'ease the burdens weighing on developing countries and threatening the developed world'. It focused on women as 'agents of change' in society and said that 'ignoring their health care, family planning, educational and economic needs is a major contribution to the problems of developing nations'.

The report urged law-makers, politicians, development agencies and international financial and lending institutions to adjust their policies to account better for women's needs. 'It called for changes in the laws of Third World nations to remove barriers to women's participation in society; equal pay for equal work; improvement of educational opportunities for girls; and a focus on family planning.'[6] In this blueprint for action lies the means to break the vicious cycle of disability that for so long has been the birthright of women in developing countries.

THE CRISIS AS AN OPPORTUNITY TO LEARN [*]
━━━━━━━━━━━━━━━━━━━━━━━ Erika Schuchardt

EXAMPLES FROM CONTEMPORARY DAILY LIFE
1. A non-disabled German woman goes to court because she had to share the company of disabled persons on her holiday in a holiday resort. She wins her case and is awarded damages amounting to most of her holiday expenses. The court gives the following grounds for its decision:

The mere presence of a group of at least 25 persons suffering from serious mental and physical disabilities constitutes a drawback warranting the reduction of the cost of the holiday. For sensitive persons, the enjoyment of a holiday can obviously be diminished by the presence of a group of severely disabled people. This is certainly the case if the group in question consists of deformed and mentally disturbed persons not mastering any language and one or other of whom emits inarticulate cries in an irregular rhythm and is seized by occasional fits. It is certainly desirable that the seriously disabled should be integrated into normal daily life, but certainly no travel agency can impose this on its other clients. The existence of suffering in the world is an unalterable fact but the complainant's desire at least to be spared the sight of it on holiday cannot be gainsaid.
[JUDGEMENT OF THE CIVIL DIVISION OF THE REGIONAL COURT, FRANKFURT-ON-THE-MAIN, GERMANY, 25 FEBRUARY 1980. NO. 24]

2. A mother, a psychotherapist, states:
Having a disabled child can place so great a burden on the parents and make such unceasing demands on them [the writer is the mother of two disabled children] that they, the mother especially as the parent most directly affected, no longer see any way out. They may deliberately seek death for themselves and their disabled child, because they believe they can no longer sustain this lifelong

---

[*] Dr Schuchardt prepared this article while with the Department of Pedagogy, University of Hanover, Federal Republic of Germany, 1981.

burden and also perhaps because they have received too little help.
[SILVIA GÖRRES, FEDERAL REPUBLIC OF GERMANY]

3. An Indian woman doctor, speaking of her paraplegia, which was caused by a traffic accident, declares:

Fate, life, God – call it what you will – it wasn't fair! ... It would have been far better if I had died instead of being only half-alive. Job in the Old Testament knew what suffering was. He had learned to say: 'If He slay me, I will wait for Him.' That wasn't all that difficult; I would gladly accept being slain. But what I have to learn to say is: 'If He slay me not ...'
[MARY VERGHESE, INDIA]

4. In a seminar session in which non-disabled children and their parents participate, a non-disabled (still unafflicted) German mother says:

I am here today because I enjoy it! But to tell the truth, I was afraid to come. I wouldn't have come had I not known Mrs Schuchardt from other seminars and if she hadn't encouraged us personally to take part in the joint seminars with parents of disabled children. You know, I once had an experience when Bettina was just a tiny tot. We were in the playground; Bettina was playing in the sandpit and I was sitting on the bench. Suddenly I noticed she was playing with a child who was quite obviously mentally handicapped. I was afraid, really afraid. I didn't know what to do. It also passed through my mind that it could be contagious, that it could be passed on. Perhaps the child was vicious! I certainly didn't know this! I just picked Bettina up from the sandpit and went away!
[ROSWITA BRAUN, FEDERAL REPUBLIC OF GERMANY]

WOMEN IN THE FOREFRONT

These life situations indicate, surprisingly, that the reporters are almost invariably women. A number of statistics illustrates the preponderant role of women in efforts to deal with the crisis of disability. A perusal of the autobiographies of persons afflicted by disability reveals that about three-quarters of some 80 life stories written between 1900 and 1981 in German and English were written by women whose role was either that of the person directly afflicted with disability or that of the person sharing indirectly in it, the supporter or companion – whether wife, mother, sister, social worker or woman specialist. Male autobiographies, on the contrary, were not only in the minority but also were rarely written by men occupying the role of companion to a disabled person or persons. If we look in the secondary literature about crises or suffering and the *via dolorosa*, or on the meaning of suffering, we find that such publications were written almost exclusively by men. As reflected in the primary and secondary literature therefore, the situation is as follows:

● In the primary literature it is mostly women who, on the basis of their own experience and first-hand knowledge, describe how they coped with their crises, that is, with their suffering not only as those personally afflicted with disability but also as those accompanying a disabled person. (Of the 80 biographies examined, 64 are by women, 31 of them mothers of disabled children, 25 of them disabled themselves, and 8 women in supportive roles.)

● In the secondary literature it is mainly men who, on the basis of theory, describe possible ways and means of dealing with crises, with the emphasis more on suffering as such, and less on the more important ability to cope with suffering.

If we approach this matter from another angle, that of the diaconal, the service-oriented branch of the Church, and try to establish the relevant facts, once again we find that women are preponderant in the daily work of dealing with the afflicted. It is hardly known that human companionship and support in diaconal work is provided almost exclusively by women. It comes perhaps as an even greater surprise to learn that it is mostly men who lay down the conditions of work in this field.

> Disability is not so much a physical condition as a psycho-social crisis for those afflicted. The victims themselves are quite clear about this:
>
> 'It isn't so much the disability which paralyses, but the thousandfold handicaps caused by society. It isn't that one is disabled but that one is *turned into* a disabled person!

The four daily life situations described above, therefore, also illustrate the impairment of the interaction between the 'afflicted' and the 'still unafflicted'. This is due on the one hand to the segregated educational system, which divides the disabled and the non-disabled from infancy to entry into working life, and on the other hand to the emphasis on performance and production in industrial societies. Two consequences follow from this:

● The more differentiated and 'perfected' a sophisticated welfare society becomes, the more intensively it pursues a policy which, in practice, actually removes its afflicted citizens from care. The disabled, the sick, the aged and the dying are handed over to the care of specialised establishments and attended to by institutions, but no longer caringly cared for. In other words, we lose the dimension of human companionship in caring solidarity.

● A society operating in this highly organised way is deprived of its neces-

sary corrective. It mistakenly believes that only the disabled are dependent persons. It fails to see that society itself is invisibly dependent on the disabled for a critique of its inhumane norms and values. In view of both our domestic social problems and the problems of the world community (for example starvation, apartheid and the gap between poor and rich), it is becoming ever clearer that the solution of these problems depends less and less on power and money and increasingly on the challenge of a radical rethinking, that is *learning*.

Hence our thesis: the disabled need society and society needs the disabled. The crisis needs to be rediscovered as an opportunity to learn!

While it is possible for the 'still unafflicted' to spend all their lives running away from burdensome situations, even though this means forfeiting in the process the opportunity to learn who they really are, it is far more difficult for disabled persons to spend their lives evading coming to terms with their disability. The question, 'How am I to live with my disability, my crisis?' can be found in all the biographies stemming from the period between 1900 and 1981. I examined what these biographies had to say about this question and discovered that all the biographers, whatever their particular disability, underwent the same learning process in three stages: from the head, via the heart, to the hand (handling!) until they achieved social integration. We have deliberately chosen to label this learning process 'crisis management' rather than 'coping with disability', as we wanted a label that would apply equally to disabled and non-disabled, to people whose personality or identity is threatened by crises that cannot be avoided. In this interaction model for social integration, therefore, crisis management is a main element.

THE EIGHT INTERLINKED OR SPIRAL PHASES OF THE LEARNING PROCESS OF CRISIS MANAGEMENT

Like the learning process in which we learn to deal with crisis, a spiral can continue indefinitely. Hence my choice of this analogy. The learning process can last a whole lifetime, since real experience depends always on our lifelong readiness to learn.

The coils of a spiral can lie flatly side by side or else be drawn asunder in a flexible manner, and this is analogous to the way in which, in the process of learning to handle a crisis, individual spiral phases can either coincide with or follow each other, and even build on one another.

To understand the process of learning to handle crises, it will be helpful if we try for a moment to enter imaginatively into the situation of an afflicted person when, for example, the doctor tells her or him: 'You have cancer ...' or 'Paraplegia is the normal outcome of your accident' or 'Your child is physically well but has a mental disability'. The receipt of such a message paralyses us as if we had been struck by lightning. Unbidden, the question poses itself: 'What really is wrong ...?' We are in the first phase of the spiral, that of uncertainty.

When the physical symptoms accumulate, there are unmistakable reactions from society, and the number of medical diagnoses increases; entry on the second phase of the spiral is inescapable: that of *certainty*. In this phase we try to reassure ourselves with the argument (Oh so familiar!): 'Yes, but ... it can't be true!' All of us know that this 'Yes, but ...' is tantamount to a straight 'No!' But this is an exact description of our situation at the end of the initial stage: our mind, or head, tells us 'It's true' but in our heart deep down we feel: 'It *can't* be true, because it *shouldn't* be true!'

The biographies in question describe graphically here how the learning process in many cases came to an abrupt end at this point. Those for whom this was true all their lives needed all their strength to evade and deny the truth they found so threatening. Often this was simply because they felt themselves to be utterly on their own and thrown back on their own resources in their efforts to learn how to cope with their crisis. They had no one to accompany them and help them to hang on in this transitional stage.

In this transitional stage, the intellectually understood message of the head very gradually percolates drop by drop to the emotional reaches of the heart. The consequence is that the emotions, which have been bottled up almost to danger point, often erupt and fly off almost uncontrollably in all directions. One can easily understand why some afflicted people, fearing instinctively at this point an uncontrollable outburst of emotion, erect a defensive wall against the insoluble personal problem and prefer to stand still and stagnate in their crash course in crisis management. They find it impossible to restrain the bitter cry: 'Why me, of all people?'

In the third phase of the spiral, that of *aggression*, the afflicted person hits out at everything and nothing. Any target will serve (family, friends, colleagues, society) because in fact the real target of this aggression is her or his disability, that is the crisis, and this, of course, is unassailable. In an analysis of 70 biographies, I found nine typical forms of aggression. I shall mention only one of these here, but this was one which was described in two-thirds of the biographies analysed. Here, aggression takes the form of wishing one's child or oneself dead. The tragic aspect of this third phase of the spiral is the vicious circle of aggression, from which escape seems impossible. The afflicted persons

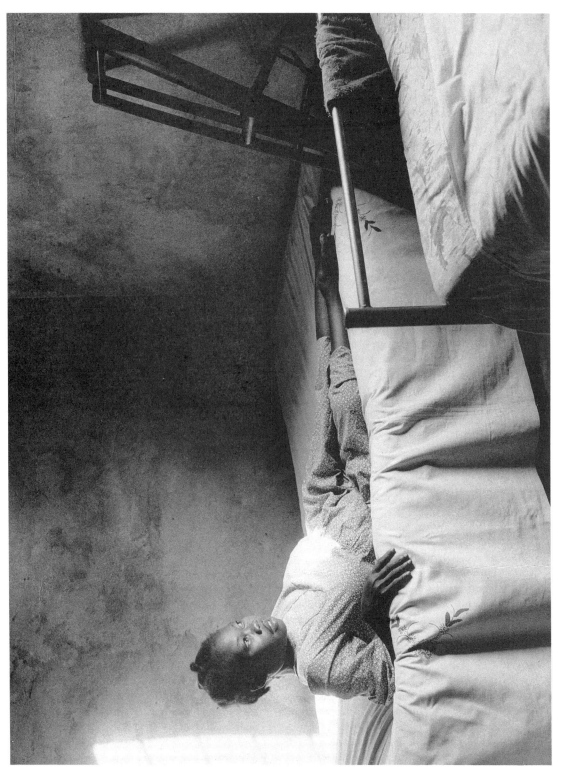

PHOTO: ANITA ANDERSSON/SHIA.

9

complains: 'Why *me?*' and becomes aggressive. The people closest at hand retort by asking: 'Why do you treat us so aggressively? It's not our fault!' and they meet aggression with aggression. This in turn confirms the afflicted person in the self-fulfilling prophecy 'Everything, everyone's against me!' and this sets the vicious circle spinning again. Only when we learn to see that each feeling of personal injury stems from a misinterpretation of the real situation is it possible for us to break out of this vicious circle.

Parallel to this phase, or building upon it, comes the fourth phase of the spiral, that of *negotiation*, with doctors, with fate, with God and the world. It may be along the lines of the question: 'If ..., then surely this means ...?' The long march through the 'world of the medical department stores' begins (the biographers report on average 23 consultations!). Alternatively, we try the search for miraculous cures (pilgrimages are described by two-thirds of the biographers). At the end of this financial and mental shopping spree, all are inevitably in a condition of material and spiritual bankruptcy. We reach the fifth phase of the spiral, that of *depression*. 'What's the use? It's all pointless!' Here again, the biographies illustrate two distinct and typical patterns of interpretation. On the one hand, there is grieving over what has now gone for good (health, the birth of a non-disabled child), in other words, what we call retrospective grief; on the other hand, there is grieving over what will presumably have to be bidden goodbye to in the future (friends, colleagues, status), in other words, anticipatory grief. Only a brief reference is possible here to the fact that an analysis of the biographies shows that two-thirds of the subjects break off their learning process at this point and for the rest of their lives persist in aggression, negotiation or depression, a condition which is equivalent to social isolation.

The sixth stage of the spiral will be described very briefly. Only a third of the biographers reach this phase: that of *acceptance*. 'Only now, for the first time do I know ... I can ...!' It is no longer a question of what has gone for good. On the contrary, it is a matter of knowing what can be achieved with what remains. For what I have is less important that what I make of what I still have. The seventh phase, that of *activity*, is the natural sequel to the sixth phase. It is now a matter of Do this ... This phase is the root of all self-help and of all pioneering groups as well as organisations which may subsequently be formed, for it culminates in the final, eighth phase of the spiral, that of *solidarity*: 'We act together ...' I begin to look away from myself and to assume my responsibilities as part of the social and collective 'We'.

Referring once again to the pyramidal character of the spiral, we find the majority of the afflicted in the initial stage and the minority in the final stage, because most – dependent only on themselves – have had to start on and persevere in this crash course of crisis management without any assistance from others.

I cannot deal here with the form taken by the learning process in the different types of disability described in the biographies, or with factors which exert an influence on it, or again with the key role played by aggression in particular.

In conclusion, two things must be said about teaching methods. The first is that in four years of practical work we have discovered that for many of those struck by disability it was helpful to have an *initial period* on their own, working directly and concretely among themselves on the clarification of their personal problems, exchanging experience, dispelling their fears and achieving stability.

Only after that was it usually possible to advance to a second stage, in which learning processes involving disabled and non-disabled people together were developed. But it is still vitally important here to keep in mind the third step: participation. In other words, the ultimate aim of educational work with disabled and non-disabled persons is to make itself superfluous. Work in target groups is never more than a bridge to education, not education itself. Target group work with disabled and non-disabled persons must not become an end in itself; it must always remain simply a means to the goal of maximum social integration. ●

THE HIDDEN 40 MILLION *

■ Sue Tuckwell

Among the many myths which shroud the subject of world poverty is the idea that the poor somehow do not suffer as the rich do. And the commonly held belief that mental illness is rare in the developing world – that life is simple but sane, lacking the mental and emotional stresses of complex modern societies – is an extreme example of that myth.

For myth it is. There is no fundamental difference between rich and poor countries in either the kind, severity or incidence of mental illness. According to the World Health Organisation, for example, there are an estimated 40 million men, women and children suffering from severe and untreated mental illness in the developing world today ...

Part of the problem is that mental illness is more nebulous. Unlike the great plagues of smallpox, cholera, malaria and hunger, mental illness offers no graspable treatment, no identifiable germ, no available vaccine, and people rarely die from it. But as Dr Abdus Sobha, consultant psychiatrist at Bangladesh's Pabna Mental Hospital says, 'The brain is as important

as the stomach and the lungs. We should not segregate this aspect of health from all others.'

More women than men suffer from mental illness in the Third World, but far more men are getting treatment.

The problem is also partly one of fear, misunderstanding and stigma – breeding an attitude of 'I don't want to know'. Many studies have been published on the effects of malnutrition on the growth of the body. But near silence reigns on the effect of malnutrition on the growth of the mind.

Obviously, there is also a perennial economic problem. Most people simply cannot afford treatment for mental illness. A study carried out at the post-graduate hospital in Dhaka, Bangladesh, shows just how élite are the psychiatric out-patients – 93 per cent of the men and 79 per cent of the women could read and write, as opposed to a national norm of 22.2 per cent – most of them male.

The average mental patient passes through a series of economic sieves, beginning with the local healers, graduating to local doctors and hospitals, and eventually passing to either the large teaching hospitals or the Pabna Mental Hospital itself. Many, many drop out along the way – for the family must make realistic decisions about how to spend a limited amount of money.

Poverty alone does not cause mental illness, but it undoubtedly makes it worse. Stress is known to precipitate emotional illness, and the rural masses in the Third World, subject to frequent bereavement, floods, fires, famines, wars, enforced migration, and rising expectations unmatched by rising incomes, would seem to be under great emotional pressure. Yet

* *New Internationalist*, January 1981. Journalist Sue Tuckwell interviewed doctors, psychiatrists and social workers in Bangladesh and Africa for this report.

little is known about their feelings and reactions.

Particularly vulnerable are the women. A pioneering study of a Bangladeshi village has put facts around that conclusion. Sixty-nine out of every 1,000 people were found to have significant psychiatric illness – but women outnumbered men, two to one. Most of them were suffering from anxiety neurosis and depressive illness.

Dhaka family planning workers unanimously agree. Most families they visited, they said, were unhappy, and the brunt of the burden fell on the women because of their total economic dependence on men, especially in times of economic crisis. A recent incident illustrates how real those fears are. A newspaper reporting a recent food shortage described how women were being divorced by their farmer husbands because there was not enough food for the whole family. This, said the writer, was very sad for the men.

Overall, it emerges clearly that more women than men are sufferers, but that far more men are getting treatment. In addition to the self-selection of mental patients, the problem finds another root in the selection of the doctors themselves. Too many doctors cannot cope with or understand the problems of the poor, or of women, because they are almost inevitably from rich backgrounds and almost invariably male.

SUPPLEMENTING THE FAMILY'S CARE

In most Third World countries, the main source of care and health for the millions who are mentally disabled is – and will continue to be – the family and the community. Fortunately, most rural societies are much more tolerant than industrialised communities of odd or eccentric behaviour, especially among the very young or the very old. And they will normally try to care for the sufferer within the family as long as is possible. The true measure of the success of mental health programmes is how effectively they supplement the family's care – by identification of disability, by drugs, by counselling, and by the teaching of simple, low-cost treatment. Another yardstick is the degree to which they reach women, children and disadvantaged groups. And a third essential criterion is cost – how cheaply can it be done, how can the maximum number of people take advantage of any service that can be provided.

Unlike smallpox, mental illness can never be eradicated. But recognition of the incidence and severity of the problem – and its effects on the quality of human life and on every other aspect of the development effort – is long overdue. ●

CARIBBEAN INTERVIEW

Susan Sygall, Mobility International

The following verbatim interview is one of several carried out during the Disabled People's International Conference on Disabled Women and Development, held in Roseau, Commonwealth of Dominica, in the Caribbean, in July 1988. The interviewee was Evincia Edwards, aged twenty-five, of St Kitts.

Q: *Evincia, what do you think are the problems of disabled women in the Caribbean?*

A: We don't get much response from society.

Q: *Tell me a little about yourself.*

A: I have one child, I am not married and am unemployed. What makes it hard is that people don't see you as a normal human being. I became blind after the doctor gave me an injection. I didn't know what was wrong. I was partially blind for a few years then became totally blind. I went to a school for blind people where I learned Braille.

Q: *What do you like about this conference?*

A: I like to meet people, like yourself. Hearing other disabled women speak gives you courage and strength.

Q: *If you could do anything in the next ten years, what would you want to do?*

A: I would like to be a leader in an organisation and help other people. I accept my disability. The problem in the Caribbean is that people don't accept their disability. I'd like to be a leader to survey and help others come out and see they are not put aside and they still are human beings and help them see the light …

Q: *There has been a lot of talk at the conference about disabled women and their relationships. What do you think?*

A: Men use you … then leave you – push you aside – they think you can't do nothing. I am surprised to hear that some disabled women are married. They say that we shouldn't be married and shouldn't have a boyfriend because we can't do nothing.

Q: *Can you change people's attitude?*

A: No, because it goes in one ear and out the other … If you want to see the building where we have school – Oh Lord have mercy – there is a hole in the floor – water dripping from the roof – the building is so old …

We have to struggle a lot – disabled people won't come out – there was someone trying to encourage a blind woman to go to school – she wouldn't go – didn't want to come out – she don't want to be disabled …

After I became disabled, I learned Braille and was encouraged … I had a teacher who encouraged me. He said, 'When you're down – you're up.' If I didn't go to school, I wouldn't. be at the conference.

We have a small disabled organisa-tion, but people don't attend the meetings so they don't do much … ●

THE IMAGE MAKERS ☐ Disabled women know about image makers – not the slick professionals who turn out personality packages to order, but society itself.

The public, in industrialised countries particularly, is brainwashed by a constant bombardment of images of the commercialised ideals of womanhood – young, beautiful, active and physically perfect – to the extent that society strips the disabled woman of her self-respect and sexuality, and regards her not as a person but as an object of charity and pity.

The disabled woman feels so stigmatised by these reactions that it becomes a major problem to cope with the social and psychological consequences. It is these that erode self-respect and motivation and foster a negative self-image of inferiority and uselessness.

The more imaginative among society's amateur image makers even hint darkly that disability is shameful, that it is somehow the fault of the disabled person for who-knows-what transgression. Even individuals with a religious orientation make a direct connection between physical perfection and spiritual beauty.

Over the years, literature has helped to perpetuate the myth that disability makes women 'different' and even menacing. The authors of such works are usually able-bodied men.

DISABLED WOMEN: PORTRAITS IN FICTION AND DRAMA*
Deborah Kent

Disabled since birth, I was in my teens

* Condensed from Michelle Fine and Adrienne Asch (eds.), *Women with Disabilities – Essays in Psychology, Culture and Politics*, Temple University Press, Philadelphia, USA.

when I began to realise that most novelists and playwrights agree that 'a cripple makes an indifferent heroine'. In the hunger for role models I searched everything I read for the woman I might some day hope to become. Over and over again, I read of graceful, dexterous, bright-eyed girls, dazzling dancers with flashing repartee, girls whose physical perfection was never questioned. They agonised over which of their numerous suitors to accept, or, if the drive for independence ran strong, they spurned all of their admirers and found fulfilment in high adventure or a challenging career.

What would have happened, I wondered, if Juliet had been blind? Would Romeo still have deemed her worthy of his love? Would Darcy have appreciated Elizabeth Bennett's wit if she had had a disfigured face? Would Emma Bovary have chafed under the yoke of married life if she had walked with a limp?

> ... the literary image of the disabled woman may influence the way disabled women are seen and judged in real life.

I longed to find proof that disability need not bar me from all of the pleasures and perils that other girls regarded as their birthright. I needed confirmation that somehow, despite society's prevailing negative attitudes, I could manage to hold on to good feelings about myself and explore a full range of options in life. Relatives and counsellors mouthed reassurance, but the few disabled women I met frightened me, with their narrow, isolated lives. And the disabled women I encountered in my reading, when I found them at all, were little consolation ...

An assessment of the disabled woman's place in literature may serve as a barometer to measure how she is perceived by society. Conversely, the literary image of the disabled woman may influence the

way disabled women are seen and judged in real life ...

Disabled women may have particular difficulties making friends. Friendships with women peers are strikingly absent from the lives of many of the disabled women in literature. In a few instances, the author simply makes no reference to friends, and the possibility remains that they hover somewhere offstage. But far more often the disabled woman is clearly isolated. She is cut off from normal interactions with other women by emotional barricades erected by herself and by the people around her.

Marriage is the ultimate goal for the unmarried woman in most works, to be single is to be an old maid – economically dependent, socially ostracised and emotionally unfulfilled.

In a number of novels and plays, disabled women do develop relationships with men. Ironically, the woman herself often strives to raise doubts in the mind of her lover. If she truly loves him, she must protect her man from taking on an intolerable burden. At the same time, in testing a man's commitment she is attempting to protect herself from the pain of future rejection.

DISABILITY, AN OVERWHELMING ISSUE

Nearly all the relationships I have described turn upon the woman's disability. If she is an isolate, deemed unqualified by men, it is because she is disabled. Potential mates doubt her competence to tend to a family. Frequently the man feels he will be diminished in the eyes of others if he can acquire only a substandard partner. If on the other hand a man finds the disabled woman attractive, it is because her disability draws him to her, making her mysterious, heroic, or appealingly vulnerable. In either case, disability looms as an overwhelming issue for the men in most of these works. They may be repelled or attracted to the disabled woman, or struggle with both feelings at once. But the woman's disability is nearly always seen as her first and most salient attribute.

The disabled woman is often seen from the outset as a victim. She is not acted upon by random circumstance, but is physically damaged by someone in her life, most commonly by a man. This image of the disabled woman as victim serves to heighten the sense that she is inadequate and helpless, more vulnerable than her non-disabled peers.

In many instances, the disabled woman is little more than a metaphor through which the writer hopes to address some broader theme. Her disability may stand for helplessness, innocence, or blighted opportunity.

Does art imitate life, or does life imitate art? In the case of the disabled woman, both seem to be true. Even at their best, most of these writers focus chiefly upon the most negative aspects of life as a disabled woman – the helplessness and isolation, the sense of inferiority. For many women with disabilities such a portrait is all too accurate. Yet a great number of disabled women do not fit this picture at all. Those who lead satisfying lives, thoroughly integrated into the community, are rarely found in literature. By failing to offer more positive images, these writers help to perpetuate the negative stereotypes they present. The non-disabled reader comes away from most of these works with awe and pity.

The disabled woman, searching as I did through my growing-up years, will find few positive role models in their pages. Instead, most of these novels and plays confirm our most deep-seated fears about how we appear to others and what our lives may hold. There aren't many of these characters I would like to get to know in real life; there are even fewer I

would ever want to become. ●

WHAT'S SO IMPORTANT ABOUT THE WRAPPING PAPER ON OUR SOULS?*

Mary Jane Owen, MSW

Many disabled people wonder how they will be welcomed by the membership of various churches and temples. It is unfortunately not unusual for most of us to have good people approach us with unsolicited suggestions, made on the basis of superficial information garnered from our physical imperfections. Someone who knows nothing about me except that I use a white cane as a mobility aid will startle me by approaching unexpectedly and hissing in my direction, 'If you truly believe in the Lord, He could make you see before you get to the end of the block.'

Do we really judge the status of another's soul on the basis of its container? Are the physical trappings and wrappings so indicative of one's relationship with God? It often seems we evaluate the depth of religious belief on the basis of bodily perfection. We seem to assume, with Job's friends, that if one is 'right' with the Lord, there is no excuse for having either boils or more severe physical flaws. There is clear evidence that many individuals with a wide range of religious orientations make a direct connection between physical perfection and spiritual beauty. It seems small wonder that many disabled people are discouraged from looking for a religious home.

DISTURBING EXAMPLE

I observed the following example several months ago, in an upper-income suburb of a very cosmopolitan urban centre. A

---

* From *Rehabilitation Gazette*, Vol. 27, No. 2, 1986.

series of healing services was being conducted by a visiting priest who was warmly introduced and endorsed by the local bishop. The service began with simpleprayers and unison singing, but within a short time became more emotionally complex and contradictory. The priest asserted that only the devil within us prevents each and every one from immediately acquiring a perfect body. After several hours, he ordered the doors and windows to be thrown open so that those of us with the mark of the devil could more easily throw him out.

At this point, my friends and I became aware of two individuals in front of us. A young child was sitting in a wheelchair and my friends told me she obviously had some neuromuscular condition that prevented her from holding up her head. Her chin rested on her chest and her arms lay limply in her lap. She had been pushed there by her father, who now stood over her loudly demanding, 'Come on honey, you know you love Jesus. Just get up now … Come on, all you have to do is believe. Put all the evil thoughts out of your mind right now and pray harder to the Lord to forgive you for your evil ways.'

The father became more frantic, apparently aware that others might believe his family guilty of various transgressions because his child had such obvious defects. He called one of the ushers to help pull the confused girl out of her chair and on to her feet. Tears filled my eyes as I thought of the pain and anguish that were being added to this family's life. The challenge of a disabled child might seem to be strain enough, but it appeared their church and religious beliefs were adding to that stress. My friends and I had been to services that emphasised the calm healing of the soul. We believed in the miracle of the Eucharistic Feast, but there was something terribly wrong in what was being played out in front of us. We left

during the next hymn, not willing to disturb the service, but each of us in moral turmoil.

> The priest asserted that only the devil within us prevents each and every one from immediately acquiring a perfect body.

Recently, I was asked to address the coffee hour at my church about accessibility. There was a flurry of interest in modification because the old architectural drawings, which illustrated the planned extensions to the present building, were discovered and displayed.

I talked about the problems of architectural accessibility and used a bit of acceptable rhetoric about attitudinal barriers. But a dark shadow seemed to lurk at the back of all the practical suggestions about building and creating an hospitable environment. It began to dawn on me that it is not just ignorance about the creative aspects of accessible design that prevents people from giving up some of their ideas about religious architecture. Perhaps there is a widely perceived need to retain an inaccessible sanctuary – a retreat from all that is 'flawed'.

There are questions that those of us involved within the conceptual framework of the healing community need to explore but that we avoid because the implications are too threatening to our idealism. Some disability scholars are suggesting that the resistance to making our society accessible to the whole range of disabled and elderly people may best be explained by acknowledgement that we truly hate to be reminded of our own frailty and vulnerability. This strong negative association gets intertwined with a view of the person who, because of his or her disability, reminds all of us of the end of youth and robust health. By labelling disabled people as being in some manner responsible for their condition, we can separate ourselves from the fear that it might happen to us.

As a child, it struck me that one of my teachers actually must have decided to be so old. In retrospect, thirty years seemed about as old as one could get and, in my child's mind, I could not believe it would happen to me unless I became careless and let it happen. It is only a short step from such a view to making that judgement of the frail elderly, and if it is true for the difficulties brought by age, we can certainly begin to associate it with other physical disabilities.

Does this sort of mental process explain why it has been theologically convenient to associate evil and failure to 'get right with God' and the stubborn refusal of the 'flawed' to accept the miracle of a physical cure? Will exploration of these questions lead to better control over such fear?

A friend of mine who uses a motorised wheelchair and who is also becoming increasingly blind and deaf has a charming wit and a healthy approach to her religion's view on healing. She has always felt sure that the major reason Jesus spent so much time healing people of physical ills was because that was the only way He could seem to get people's attention. When He went on talking of His Father's Kingdom on earth in what seemed like abstract terms, His words did not excite His listeners as much as when He would simply zap someone into physical perfection. We are preoccupied with how we look today, but it seems obvious to me that people in Jesus's time were also very much concerned about not being seen as handicapped.

I don't think it matters a bit to God what our 'packaging' looks like. We were told as children that He loves the red and the brown, the black and the white, the old and the young. Yet we grow up with this undercurrent of belief that the form of our bodies is so important. Our souls are a mutual gift from and to the Lord. What's in the package doesn't get its value by how it happens to be wrapped.

When a congregation accepts the reality that members of its religious family still need to be welcomed into its buildings even when they become flawed, then God's love is surely shown through that caring. When we feel comfortable about the oncoming frailty of those we already know, we can take the risk to reach out to the stranger who is different in ways that puzzle us. We may intellectually wish to remove the barriers to full participation in the worship of our congregation, but first we may have some very human fears to explore, with respect and consideration for the basis of the terrors that keep us from fulfilling the idealistic goals of a healing community. ●

1 Susan R. Hammerman, 'Women and disability', Rehabilitation International Conference on Women with Disabilities, New York, February 1986.
2 Dr Fatima Shah, 'Issues concerning women with disability', Disabled Persons International Seminar, Seoul, Republic of Korea, 1986.
3 Excerpts from the paper by Dr Fatima Shah presented at the Seminar to Review Achievements at the Midpoint of the United Nations Decade of Disabled Persons, Bangkok, Thailand, June 1987.
4 Balakushna Venkatesh, Beacon, newsletter of the Divine Light Trust for the Blind, October 1988.
5 'Women and disabilities: a national forum', in Entourage Magazine, autumn 1988.
6 Jule Sell, 'UN Fund urges investment in women', International Herald Tribune, 17 May 1989.

2 PREVENTION – BREAKING THE VICIOUS CIRCLE

Preventing disability is easier and cheaper than rehabilitating its victims. Measures can be taken to break a vicious circle of disability stemming from malnutrition and untreated curable diseases which adds generation after generation of Third World women to the army of the disabled. A positive first step, which can serve as a major global preventive effort, is a change in the status of all women.

PREVENTION OF DISABILITY is usually easier, cheaper and certainly more desirable than rehabilitating its victims.

The fact that most disabilities can be prevented is cold comfort indeed for more than 500 million people in the world today who suffer from physical, mental or sensorial disabilities. But timely preventive measures can begin to thin the future ranks of the world's vast army of disabled, now estimated at some 10 per cent of the global population.

THE PRE-EMPTIVE STRIKE ☐ Disability is no respecter of persons – it can strike anyone, anywhere and at any time – but it strikes often the very poor, the malnourished, the illiterate. This means that women in rural and urban slum areas of developing countries are at greatest risk. Born into poverty, many of these women soon fall victim to malnutrition, poverty's deadly offspring and the principal single cause of disability. Over 100 million people are currently disabled as a result of malnutrition.

Among the major disabling conditions that women in developing countries suffer from are iron deficiency anaemia and chronic infectious pelvic disease. The anaemic condition, which is often complicated by other health problems, reduces the energy level of women, sometimes to the point that they are unable to carry out simple physical activities such as cooking or caring for children. Chronic infections in the pelvis also reduce a woman's energy level, but in addition they can cause disabling back pain. In many cases, they also cause complications during pregnancy and childbirth.

Respiratory diseases similarly count among the major disabling conditions. Chronic malnutrition, which often underlies these conditions, weakens the general state of health, making women more susceptible and less able to recover from illnesses.

The treatment for these debilitating conditions can be relatively simple if they are detected early and treated properly. But many poor women in developing countries do not receive early diagnosis and care. When the conditions become chronic they are complicated by other health problems and become increasingly difficult to treat.

In most developing countries, it is the women who grow, prepare and preserve the food, yet they may be the last to profit from their efforts. In societies where it is considered that women make little economic contribution, nutrition of the male members of the family is given first priority – a baby girl often receives only the food left by her father and brothers. When food is scarce, women and female children may receive little or no food.

Because of vitamin A deficiency in their diet, thousands of children go blind every year.

The result of such situations is that little

girls are more susceptible than boys to diseases and infections. Chronic respiratory or gastro-intestinal infections reduce a child's energy level just as they do in adults. In addition, malnourished children suffer from a diminished rate of physical and mental development. Malnourishment, which includes lack of vitamin A, can cause blindness in children. In some societies, girls are more likely than boys to suffer from these disabling conditions, which may continue to affect them throughout their lives.

One key focus should therefore be on preventive measures that concern health care. Immunisation programmes, access to safe drinking-water and proper sanitation can halt the spread of contagious and disabling diseases. A handful of green vegetables every day would be enough to save the eyesight of some 250,000 children who go blind every year because their diet lacks vitamin A. The elimination of occupational hazards such as unprotected machinery, exposure to toxic chemicals, excessive noise and vibration and insufficient light or ventilation can minimise risks to workers' health – especially for pregnant women – and reduce the number of disabling work-related accidents.

Even routine household chores can be potentially lethal. Awareness among women of the need for safety measures in the home could reduce disability among themselves and family members. Cooking with an open fire is an undoubted risk. Safe stoves and safe working equipment can help prevent disability. Leaving dangerous substances, such as gasoline and agricultural chemicals, within the reach of children provides the ingredients for serious accidents that could be prevented.

But the prevention of disability can be successful only if the community recognises the need for prevention. Awareness of this need may be raised by disabled persons and other concerned individuals.

The need for accurate data □
Involving communities in the collection of data about disability is a concrete way to start. Some are often not even aware of the frequency and extent of different types of disabilities that exist in their midst.

In conducting such surveys disability in women should receive special attention because it is usually underestimated (if reported at all), especially in rural and other poor areas. This is mainly because it is usually men who provide the information about women.

Even when they are questioned directly, women may withhold significant information about chronic conditions. The reasons are various – modesty or reluctance to admit inability or difficulty in carrying out normal duties or simply because they are ignorant of the causal relationships between behaviour and health conditions. Probably more accurate information could be obtained by women trained for the job, gathering data that would give a more realistic assessment of the incidence and types of disabilities afflicting the local female population, which would help to identify their causes.

Nutritional practices and the quality of drinking-water, for example, should be investigated if data reveal an unusually high number of sick or disabled persons in the community, especially children.

Inadequate pre-natal care, including malnutrition, too many pregnancies too early and too often, harmful traditional practices, such as female circumcision – any or all of these could underlie a pattern of children born with congenital deficiencies.

Such information can serve a preventive function, but only when health care is available. Even primary health care is not possible without community programmes to train health, social welfare and education workers.

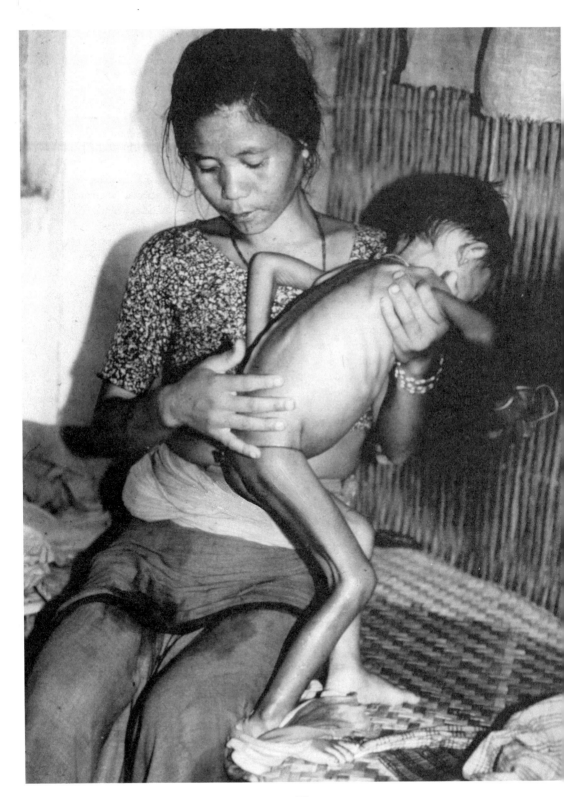

20

But prevention of disability is not a matter of health care alone – it is more complex. No vaccine exists that can immunize against hunger or malnutrition. No substitute exists for safe drinking-water, which is currently not available to 50 per cent of the world's population. Wars and other violence easily escape any net of preventive measures against disability.

Economic, social, political, cultural and attitudinal factors play a considerable role in the incidence and extent of disability. Preventive measures should therefore include not only measures that have an immediate impact but also programmes that are aimed at long-range socio-economic, structural and attitudinal changes. Governmental and non-governmental agencies alike have a moral responsibility if not to initiate, at least to encourage and support preventive activities such as immunisation programmes that can significantly reduce impairment.

Several United Nations agencies are active in the prevention of disabilities. The World Health Organisation (WHO) promotes prevention through its Primary Health Care programme. The United Nations Children's Fund (UNICEF) has a special programme for the prevention of disability among women and children. The ILO assists countries in reducing accidents and improving health in the workplace.

IMPACT, a special initiative sponsored by the United Nations Development Programme (UNDP), WHO and UNICEF, was created for one purpose: to prevent disabilities. IMPACT has established foundations in a number of countries where government and non-governmental efforts are combined for special emphasis on the prevention of diseases or conditions that can be avoided or mitigated and that could lead to blindness, deafness, physical disability or mental impairment.

Lack of iodine is the chief cause of preventable mental deficiency in the world.

WHO works with national ministries of health to develop comprehensive health services with an emphasis on prevention of disease and the promotion of health. Special programmes include maternal and child health, control of diarrhoeal disease, immunisation, prevention of blindness and deafness, control of leprosy and injury prevention.

UNICEF's disability prevention programme focuses on two of the most common nutritional deficiencies: lack of vitamin A (a major cause of blindness), and lack of iodine (the cause of goitre and cretinism and which may also contribute to deaf-mutism and neuromotor impairment. It is estimated that about 800 million people are at risk, and cretinism affects about 3 million. More than 50 per cent of these live in Southeast Asia and more than 80 per cent in Asia as a whole, but there are also important affected areas in Latin America and Africa.

UNICEF has been assisting in iodine deficiency studies and control programmes in Bhutan, Bolivia, India, Indonesia, Nepal, Pakistan and Peru. Iodine deficiency is usually controlled through iodisation of the local salt supply. UNICEF carries out and supports other measures to prevent disability including simple rehydration methods to control diarrhoea in children, training programmes for women in the prevention and early detection of childhood disabilities, and programmes for the prevention and cure of leprosy and the prevention of disability through immunisation, particularly against polio.

Women's groups can help ☐
Women's groups can be very effective, from community to national level, in stimulating action for the prevention of

disabilities. They may start in their own communities by gathering information about disabilities and their causes. The women may then initiate the actions needed in their own communities to prevent disabilities. At the same time, they can look for other outside resources, such as district or provincial health and education services. Where services are not available, they can make their needs known to government representatives.

Those who want to help prevent disabling conditions within their communities should consider the following points:

● Clean water and sanitation prevent the spread of diseases that can cause blindness or paralysis.
● Proper nutrition prevents malnourishment, which decreases the ability of people to carry out normal activities. Proper nutrition, which includes green, leafy vegetables rich in vitamin A, can also prevent blindness in children.
● Immunisation prevents diseases that can cause paralysis, blindness, deafness or mental retardation.
● Pre-natal care promotes the health of the mother and decreases the chances that she may give birth to a child with a disability.
● Appropriate care during labour decreases the possibility of birth injuries to the baby and possibly disabling injuries, such as tears or ruptures, to the mother.
● Post-natal care for mothers and babies promotes proper nutrition, immunisation and early detection of conditions that could cause disabilities.
● Safety precautions taken within the home can prevent potentially disabling accidents.
● Safety precautions at work sites can prevent diseases and accidents that cause a variety of disabilities. These include the disabilities which result from respiratory dysfunctions, burns, amputation, paralysis, eye injury, hearing impairment, and so on.

To prevent disabilities requires the efforts of individuals, communities and governments. Ministries of health, education, labour and social services should be involved in the dissemination of information, the development of services, and the regulation of practices related to the prevention of disability and the promotion of health and safety. Communities must take action to educate members about the causes and prevention of disabilities, and to establish health and safety measures in the community. Individuals must also take responsibility for making use of the information and services that are provided.

Such measures should be expanded to include provisions for a positive change in the status of women. Such a change, besides improving the situation of women with disabilities, can serve as an important global preventive effort.

The link between disability and low status □ The low status of women is detrimental not only to them but also to the entire human community. Society cannot afford to continue to disregard and denigrate the role, tasks and services performed by women, on which its well-being so heavily depends. To devalue these tasks and services leads to women being neglected. Appropriate technology, for example, is seldom developed for tasks performed by women, an omission that results in prolonged working hours, fatigue, diseases and disability of women with a consequent adverse effect on the entire family.

The education of women could significantly reduce the frequency of disability, which is notably higher among illiterate women than among those who have received even a basic education.

To perpetuate the status of women as second-class citizens is to maintain obstacles on the road to development and hamper efforts to achieve progress, be it economic, social or political.

TRADITIONAL PRACTICES THAT INFLICT DISABILITY*
Berhane Ras-Work

In most developing countries, women are subjected to harmful traditional practices that can inflict various kinds of serious disabilities.

Some of these practices so far identified are female circumcision, early childhood marriage and early pregnancy, and skin burning. These practices are prevalent and millions of women and children suffer from them.

Female circumcision alone is performed in twenty-five African countries as well as in Indonesia, Malaysia and Yemen. This involves cutting away all or part of the external genital organs. The degree of operation varies from excision to infibulation.

The complications resulting from this operation are haemorrhage, infection, tetanus, keloid formation, fistula cases (causing incontinence), obstructed labour and even death. These very serious consequences have been documented in the reports of the WHO Khartoum Seminar in 1979, the NGO Working Group Seminar in Dakar in 1984, and the Inter-African Committee Seminar in Addis Ababa in 1987. The reasons advanced for the existence and persistence of this practice include: to ensure chastity; to conform with religious beliefs; initiation rites and aesthetic considerations.

In spite of the seriousness of the problem it has received very little attention from governments and remains shrouded in indifference on the part of policy-makers.

Female circumcision is a silent emergency that continues to menace at least 80 million women and young girls. Injuries resulting from femal circumcision, childhood marriage and early pregnancy, malnutrition and frequent childbearing have been identified as the main causes of obstetric fistulae, a disability with devastating social and psychological consequences. Women sufferers are often deserted by their husbands and shunned by their communities and thus forced into social isolation.

A ban on childhood marriages and injurious traditional practices, improved nutrition for young girls and the introduction of effective family planning are among the recommendations to prevent obstetric fistulae. For those women already afflicted, information on access to treatment and cure of the condition should be made available.

The only concrete efforts to stop harmful traditional practices are undertaken by non-governmental organisations. The Geneva-based NGO Working Group on traditional practices has been dealing with the issue since 1977. It sends study missions and initiates programmes of education and sensitisation. It lobbies at appropriate international meetings in order for the problem to gain the commitment of governments. In 1984 in Dakar, it organised a regional seminar on traditional practices in collaboration with the government of Senegal, WHO and UNICEF. This proved to be an appropriate African forum where the issue was brought into the open and discussed. The men and women present at the seminar unanimously decided to work to abolish the practices of female circumcision, early childhood marriage and early pregnancy, nutritional taboos and the forced-feeding of women.

---

* Berhane Ras-Work is President of the Inter-African Committee on Traditional Practices, Addis Ababa.

23

The Inter-African Committee on Tradition-al Practices Affecting the Health of Women and Children (IAC) was created to follow up the implementation of programmes.

Since its creation, the IAC has endeav-oured to mobilise public opinion against harmful practices. It conducts grassroots education campaigns involving religious leaders, traditional birth attendants (TBAs), women leaders, health agents, doctors and nurses. It organises seminars, training sessions and workshops for identi-fied target groups. It produces visual aids, leaflets and posters. All its activities are carried out by national affiliates or other interested local partners.

Cautious educational campaigns have shown positive and encouraging results. More and more men and women are becoming aware of the problem. But its magnitude is such that the efforts of NGOs alone will not be able to solve it: commitment and action on the part of governments are necessary.

African women have addressed collec-tive appeals to governments to take action towards the total abolition of harmful practices such as female circumcision. These collective appeals were made during the conference of the UN Decade for Women, the NGO Forum, and at the IAC regional seminar in 1987. The women are still awaiting replies in the form of policies and concrete action. ●

REHABILITATION, EDUCATION, EMPLOYMENT – ELUSIVE GOALS

The facilities, encouragement and general support that are accorded to disabled men in their struggle for integration into the mainstream of society are too often not available or available only with difficulty to women with disabilities. Most rehabilitation services are male-oriented – education is an uphill struggle for disabled women and society seems to take for granted that disabled men should be employed but that disabled women are to remain dependent throughout their lives.

COMMUNITY INVOLVEMENT is adding a new and badly needed dimension to rehabilitation, especially in developing countries where 80 per cent of the world's disabled live but where only 10 per cent of all rehabilitation resources can be found.

Community-based rehabilitation services... should be established with urgency... Through these services, women with disability can be reached and along with the rendering of rehabilitation services can be trained to become contributing members of society.[1]

REHABILITATION – THE TREND TO-WARDS COMMUNITY INVOLVE-MENT □ In Botswana, a community-based rehabilitation programme is already having a great impact:

in particular, in respect to females who are disabled, as they benefit from the services of medical rehabilitation, education and vocational training right at the level where the majority of them live. Due to the community approach, attitudes in the rural areas have changed and even women with disabilities nowadays can be seen participating in family and community activities.[2]

Community-based rehabilitation is a trend now being promoted by many international organizations. For example, WHO is assisting in the development of...

the delivery of rehabilitation services at all levels, from the community where people with disabilities live, to the national level where the most specialised services are available. The crucial component of community-based rehabilitation, however, is the existence of services available in their community. A person with a disability undergoes training to perform daily activities such as eating, dressing, communicating, moving around and taking part in school, work and social activities. A family member is preferred as the trainer, but a community worker for community-based rehabilitation is available to supervise the training programme.[3]

> While family members are preferred as trainers of disabled persons, other services must be available at community level.

Such programmes involve family and community members so that those closest to disabled people can participate in improving the conditions of their lives. They also rely on locally produced appliances and technical aids that can increase the mobility and productive capacity of a person with a handicap. These devices are made of materials such as bamboo, rattan, leather and wool, which are readily available locally, rather than of costly imports which are often inappropriate for use under difficult conditions and whose repair requires repetition parts or profes-

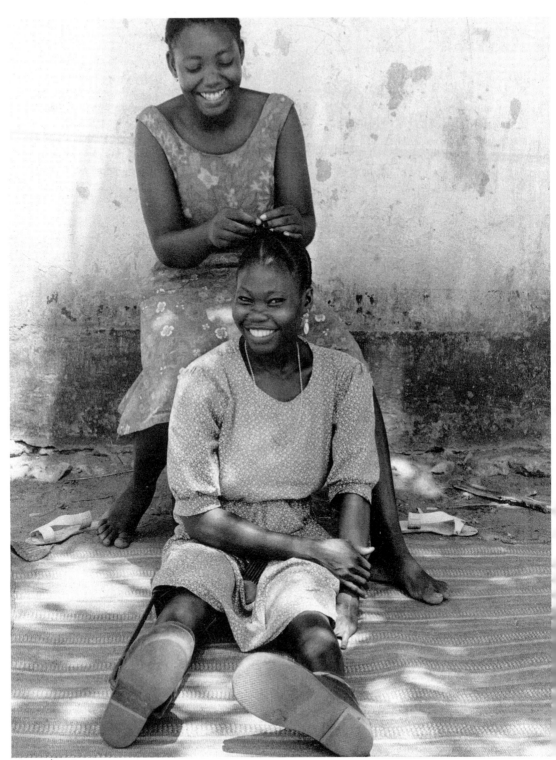

Debora and friend, Tanzania.

sional skills that are either unavailable or simply too expensive.

Community-based rehabilitation seems to fit the needs of women with disabilities much more than other approaches in rehabilitation because these women usually have a poor educational background. The majority of disabled women in developing countries live in rural areas for whom institutional rehabilitation services are neither suitable nor accessible. Moreover, there is a growing tendency to avoid the creation of large rehabilitation institutions, which are costly to run and not particularly effective in meeting the needs of disabled people to participate in the economy and in society. They also serve further to isolate disabled persons from family and community.

Unsolved problems ☐ This is not to say that community-based rehabilitation is the complete answer to all problems, nor does the concept meet with universal agreement. As yet, it is very much in the process of evolving, with some critics still not entirely satisfied.

Of the unsolved problems the most serious is to find, recruit, train, compensate, supervise and retain the field personnel needed to stimulate, motivate, train and supervise the people in the communities. Examples of apparent success have depended on infusions of external aid in the forms of both people and money – and transportation, which is often the key to making the system work. Manuals are helpful in some situations as training tools but, when dealing with pre-literate people or even those who are not accustomed to acting on the basis of books, they are not sufficient. Trained, supervised and available community-level workers are essential.

Closely linked to the above is the

problem, or complex of problems, inherent in the policies of governments.

The resources to place in the field a network of trained personnel and to maintain, transport and supervise them so that they can service the entire population must come from governments. Without the necessary governmental policies, funding budgets and machinery, activation of an effective service system based on community-level action will always be limited to test areas and experimental action.

Programmes are called 'second class' services and are seen to be 'limiting' rather than 'liberating' as they disregard individual potential.

There can be no higher aim for a government than to plan the systematic development and maintenance of a balanced network of facilities and services ranging from the highly specialised, as needed, to the outreach of workers in the most remote villages. None has such a plan, no aid-giving agencies are advising the preparation of such plans.[4]

But while community-based rehabilitation has been criticised as a strategy of 'second class' service reserved for the poor, it has also been pointed out that an estimated 70 per cent of the people who could benefit from rehabilitation services could have their needs met at community level. The majority would otherwise have no hope of obtaining help during their lifetime from institution-based programmes.

Another criticism that has been levelled at community-based programmes is that they can be 'limiting' rather than 'liberating'. This occurs where success is measured by how many new tasks a disabled person has been 'trained' to perform, with little or no notice taken of the individual's preferences and unique potential, especially when the individual is a woman.

This lack of attention to personal wishes and ability is not confined to community-based programmes. In the United States of America (USA) it was found that institution-based rehabilitation for disabled men featured job counselling, job training and job placement, while rehabilitation for women with disabilities was focused on physical therapy. 'Policies developed for the vocational rehabilitation of disabled women have to take account of the whole of the lives they actually lead.'[5]

Rural women's isolation from services

□ Most women with disabilities in Asia, Africa, Latin America, and the Middle East do not benefit from any kind of vocational rehabilitation because they live in areas where there is no transport to such services and also because of the over-protectiveness of parents or the incompatibility of rehabilitation goals with family tradition. While training opportunities for women, in general, are starting to be established in developing countries, none of the 55 successful projects for women in Africa involved women with disabilities.

When questioned, the participants said that the organizers did not think there were any disabled women in their areas, that the schemes were not relevant or that to include disabled women would present additional problems.[6]

Examples of the results of official policies emerge clearly in excerpts from some country position papers, presented at an ILO meeting in Harare, on developing programmes to aid disabled women and female children in Southern Africa.[7]

Malawi. Vocational rehabilitation is available in training centres which at present have a capacity of about 300; 70 places are occupied by women. A training programme for disabled children and their mothers is in existence and a new vocational rehabilitation centre for both men and women offers training which includes metal/woodwork, tailoring and domestic skills.

Swaziland. Vocational training possibilities for disabled women outside rehabilitation centres – where at present 30 per cent of the enrollees are female with a disability – are very limited. The present vocational rehabilitation programmes are not particularly geared toward disabled women. Programmes do, however, exist to train women for self-employment, and the involvement of women with disability in these programmes could be possible.

Tanzania. So far, efforts to involve women with disabilities in vocational training programmes have failed, as the place and role of women in general, and of disabled women in particular, are supposed to be in the home. This attitude seems to be even more prevalent in rural than in urban areas.

Zambia. Because women with disabilities are multiply handicapped in that they are female, illiterate, disabled and live in rural areas, they do not benefit as much from the available rehabilitation services as they legally could.

Zimbabwe. After national independence, priority was given to the rehabilitation of both male and female ex-combatants and war victims. Not surprisingly, existing services were overwhelmed. Further research is needed to provide a clear picture of the position of disabled women.

Follow-up action generated by the Harare meeting included a new three-year project – 'Improved livelihood for disabled women: a regional promotional programme for Southern African countries' – implemented by the ILO and financed by the Federal Republic of Germany; this project got underway in late 1989.

It has been estimated that in Southern Africa there are about 1 million disabled women, who have a total of about 4 million dependants. Many of these women have been abandoned by their husbands, and most live in abject poverty in rural areas.

The new ILO project will promote the participation of disabled women in projects and programmes for non-disabled women, and will work in close co-operation with community resources, general developmental programmes as well as rehabilitation centres in order to upgrade the education and skills of women with disabilities. In addition, it will ensure that they are provided with mobility aids and other assistive devices as required, and it will supply seed money for a revolving loan scheme.

Focusing on disabled women in Botswana, Lesotho, Swaziland, Zambia and Zimbabwe, the project's aim is to gain equal economic opportunities and improved living standards for women with disability, who are seen to have the potential to become economically competitive. One of the primary means toward achieving this goal is the creation of national networks of programmes and resources involved in the integration of disabled women, which could operate independently after the project ends.

The social and vocational well-being of blind persons, however, has preoccupied national and international organisations of and for the blind for some time, and special efforts have been made to overcome the discrimination and prejudices facing blind women in the Third World.

Asia has been especially active in this field; various agencies have organised leadership training courses and vocational training and rehabilitation programmes for blind girls and women.

In Singapore, Hong Kong, Thailand and

the Philippines, all trained, blind female telephone operators find jobs, whilst in Pakistan, some 20 blind women with Masters' degrees are employed as lecturers and teachers in sighted colleges and blind schools. In Bangladesh, India, Indonesia, Pakistan, the Philippines and Thailand, blind women are working as factory hands, packers, cane-weavers, doll and paper flower makers, knitters and dressmakers. Some educated blind women in India and the Philippines are employed as social workers and musicians; a few are receptionists and dictaphone typists. Jobs as Braille transcribers and handicraft teachers are also available to qualified blind women.

Information-based rehabilitation*

□ Although the majority of women with disabilities or care-giving women have no access to professional rehabilitation networks, many do have regular access to radio broadcasting. They are therefore able to have access to the audible content of rehabilitation work and counselling. Audible content alone, while a poor substitute for a skilled counsellor or instructor, would be much better than nothing and if governments would take a decision to make use of it, work could begin relatively quickly and easily, with an extremely small unit cost. Whilst a radio broadcast may only be 5 per cent as effective as a three-dimensional therapist, it can reach a target several hundred thousand times greater for a modest initial investment, can repeat at comparatively very low cost and can change attitudes by involving women with disabilities and enabling them to speak for themselves.

As these women increasingly shared knowledge and skills with other workers, the rehabilitation field as a whole could be seen as an information system, storing knowledge and skills in various ways, giving access and permitting transmission by

---

* This section was contributed by Mike Miles, who worked to develop community-based programmes in Pakistan.

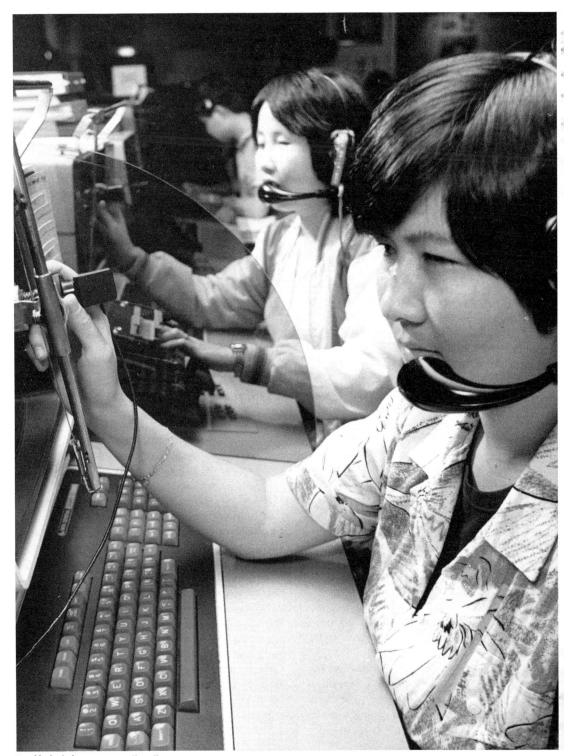

Two blind telephone operators, Hong Kong.

various media, some giving greater quality and immediacy, others giving greater coverage.

To take up the information challenge is not an easy option, but for the majority of women with disabilities or care-giving women in the world, it is the only option that could, by the year 2000, add modern formal rehabilitation science to whatever they have discovered for themselves. In this potential admixture of information for and by women with disabilities lies the greatest hope for their future.

EDUCATION – AN UPHILL STRUGGLE
☐ In Asia, 66 per cent of all women are illiterate, and in Africa, the proportion is 85 per cent. With such high rates of illiteracy among women in general in developing countries, the chances for disabled women to get an education are practically nil.

In every economic setting, children of literate women have a better chance of survival than those of illiterate women and research now suggests that the education of girls is one of the best health investments which any developing country can make. Yet two out of every three illiterate people in the world are women.'

Dr Fatima Shah, Founder President of the Pakistan Association for the Blind, has been quoted as saying that in an average Asian home, especially in rural areas, disabled girls are 'just left to exist in a confined area of the house. Very few, if any, have the chance for any kind of education.'

Two out of every three illiterate people in the world are women.

In societies where the education of women is considered a frivolous luxury, very few people realise the value of a liter-

ate mother. If girls attend school at all, they are taken out when extra hands are needed at home – boys rarely are. 'Thus, opportunities for improving the quality of life, such as better nutrition, family planning and domestic hygiene become inaccessible to those most in need.'[10]

Two major issues concerning the education of disabled women can be identified, in developed as well as developing countries: women who are disabled have less access to educational systems than non-disabled or male counterparts; and when education is available, it perpetuates a traditionally narrow role for women.

In the United States:

School systems are described as inadequately supportive of the special needs of disabled women. For example, schools do little to foster independence and to counter the over-protectiveness of family, often fail to distinguish among disabilities and level of severity, often teachers are not adequately prepared to work with disabled students... In general, women who have disabilities receive little encouragement to continue their education... It has also been suggested that disabled women suffer from discrimination in guidance and counselling.

Access to education of disabled women is further hindered by attitudes of parental overprotection and traditional role perceptions. An interesting exception is reported in two rural areas of India. In Orissa and Maharashtra, disabled girls are viewed as less likely to marry and therefore must be educated to survive. For the most part, however, the stereotype of the passive, dependent female role is more strongly reinforced by disability, often resulting in limited achievement and motivation.'[11]

The abilities of disabled young girls and women are often underestimated. Just because a woman is confined to a wheelchair it is commonly assumed that she is best at work with her hands. Consequently, many women who are disabled spend tedious hours employed in cottage industries, in work for which little education is necessary. Very few people seem to realise that a woman who has a disability may, with the proper education, have the potential to be, for example, a good lawyer, administrator, programmer or musician.

In Japan, it was found that:

Disabled women workers with a high educational background tend to establish a unique work position and maintain the post for a long period. They find jobs in areas where they do not have to compete with the non-disabled, such as language, therapy, music and managerial skills.[12]

But people with disabilities do not always need special training. They can often readily participate in programmes for the general population – if buildings are accessible, if transportation is available and if the attitudes of the able-bodied do not discourage them from taking part. Every effort should be made to facilitate and encourage the participation of disabled people in regular education and training programmes in normal settings, using specialised institutions only when it is absolutely necessary. Even these institutions should aim at helping people who have disabilities to develop capabilities necessary for their eventual integration into the normal school system.

Are special schools needed? □ In India, it is estimated that hardly 1 per cent of women who are disabled may have had an opportunity for education in the forty years since independence. Not more than 5 per cent of disabled children have benefited from educational programmes during that period.

The desirability of maintaining special schools for disabled Indian children was recently called into question.

Special schools are a hangover of the past which looked down on disabled persons as a social scourge and hence a liability. True, special schools contributed to the educational growth of disabled children at a time when society detested disability. However, it is now time for serious thinking whether we should continue to promote special schools in our country where the disabled child does not experience the atmosphere of an open society and his non-disabled peers are denied the opportunity to develop a genuine compassion for human beings less fortunate than themselves... Rather, the special schools should be converted into resource centres to train children for integrated education, which is the best foundation for normalisation of disabled persons.[13]

The responsibilities of school systems toward disabled children were stressed in a Consultation on Special Education held by UNESCO in May 1988, to review the current situation and plan action for the period 1990–95. A summary of the report of the meeting mentions some general principles which should be considered in education for disabled children:[14]

Disabled persons are entitled to an education that is comprehensive and provides a continuity of services, from early detection and early intervention, through schooling, vocational education, independent living in the community and lifelong education. Education should respond to their specific needs rather than to their category of disability.

Responsibility for special education is the responsibility of the total education system. There should not be two separate systems of educational provision. Indeed, the wider education system itself will benefit from making the necessary modifications to accommodate the needs of disabled children.

For disabled children, early childhood

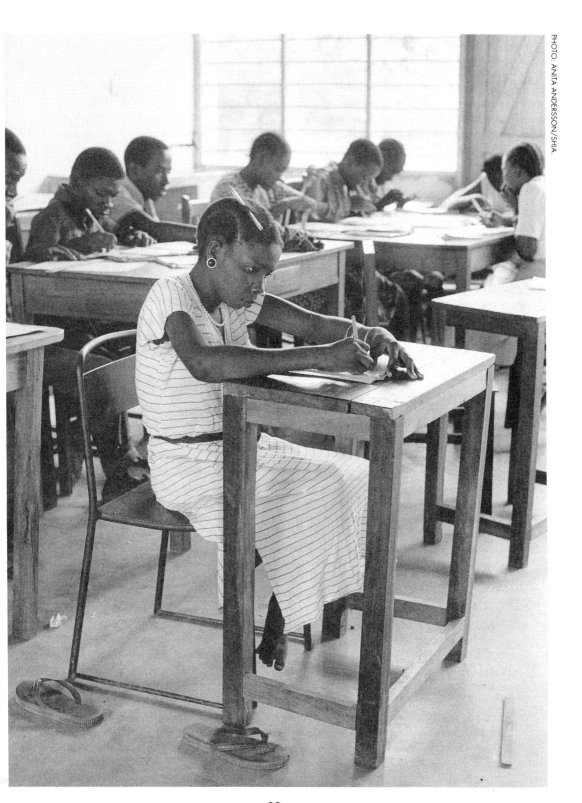

PHOTO: ANITA ANDERSSON/SHIA.

and pre-school education is critical for the development of the person's full potential. Education concerns everything that helps children to develop and early intervention is fundamentally an educative process... Parents of disabled children can play a major role in their education... Professionals impinge on the lives of disabled persons for a limited timespan and in certain contexts only. If they are to have maximum beneficial effect, their input must be integrated with the more enduring involvement of parents. Education does not end with the completion of schooling. All educational resources for disabled persons should not be expended at the pre-school and school levels. Due attention should be given to vocational education as well as adult education.

The UNESCO Consultation recognised integrated education and community-based rehabilitation as two complementary approaches in providing cost-effective and meaningful education and training for disabled persons. Both measures aim at reaching out to the greatest number of people who are disabled, and to their families.

The challenge to special schools, then, is to find ways of sharing their expertise and resources. Some have already begun to develop outreach programmes. These can entail setting up working links with neighbourhood ordinary schools where staff and pupils are shared. Some special schools act as resource centres, providing information and consultancy to local schools, organising support services for families and contributing to in-service training activities. Discharging these functions successfully requires considerable changes among special school staff. New skills must be developed and new attitudes fostered.

Special schools of the future could be very different from those that exist now. The emphasis would move away from educating limited numbers of pupils in relative isolation and towards acting as resource centres. The latter could encompass curriculum development, in-service training, the collectivon and evaluation of equipment and computer software, and specialist assessment, as well as advice and consultation on all matters relating to the education of persons with disabilities.

Special schools were a preoccupation at another 1988 meeting, the National Conference on Special Education held in Beijing, China, in November 1988. The meeting emphasised the need for compulsory education for disabled children; statistics show that this need is urgent. There are nearly 5 million disabled children in China, aged from seven to fifteen years, with visual impairment, hearing impairment or who are mentally retarded. Fewer than 6 per cent of the total are enrolled in schools.

To establish separate schools has until now been China's chief policy for the development of special education. But it has become increasingly apparent that this policy has delayed the provision of education. The conference decided that ordinary schools should include special classes for the benefit of disabled children in their neighbourhoods, while special schools should continue to serve their unique functions.

Just as one swallow does not make a summer, two conferences are by no means a global movement, but they are welcome signs that education for disabled people is a growing international concern.

FOR WHO AMONG US HAS NOT SPILLED KETCHUP*
━━━━━━━━━━━━━━━━━━━━ Lisa Blumberg

My disability was not detected in early infancy. It was only when I became a tod-

---

* Reprinted from *Rehabilitation Gazette*, Vol. 27, No. 2, 1986.

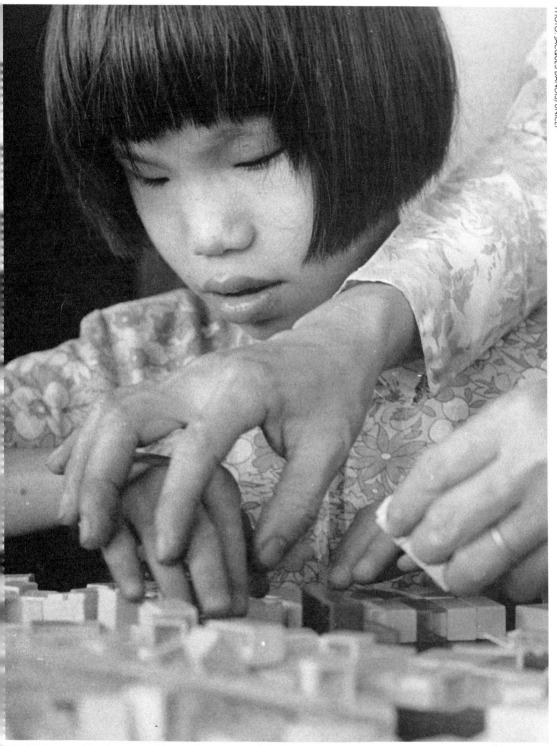

PHOTO: JACQUES DANOIS/UNICEF

A blind Vietnamese girl receives a manual dexterity lesson as part of rehabilitation.

dler who did not toddle, a wild grabber who did not grip, that the strange term athetosis was associated with me. Perhaps now, with CAT (Computerised Axial Tomography) scans, athetosis, which is an unusual form of cerebral palsy, can be spotted closer to birth. I hope not. I am sure that I benefited from those months of being treated as an ordinary baby. My mother always said that since she and my father had been caring successfully for me right along with my older brothers for quite a while before they heard the news, it was easier for them to perceive that my disability was only a small aspect of me and not my sum and substance.

A HAPPY CHILDHOOD

Although my disability affected my gait, speech, and co-ordination, few of my childhood memories are linked with being disabled. Much of the credit for this goes to my parents but at least a small part of it goes to a brilliant orthopaedist I saw just twice a year. The late Dr Sidney Keats was unusual... Unlike many orthopaedists, he avoided surgery and bracing... [his] approach was whole-person oriented. He believed that athetosis could not be cured because it was not a disease. However, just as a dancer could surpass what would otherwise be her physical potential by consistent exercise, so could I. More important, he stressed to my parents that my success in life would almost wholly depend on my being given the same opportunities for fun and learning that I would have been given had I been an ordinary child.

Dr Keats felt it was crucial for a youngster with a purely physical disability to attend regular school classes. Special education was inferior, segregated education that could handicap anyone for life. Thus, when I was six, I started first grade at the public school that my borthers attended. Most of my teachers were open-minded

and understanding. The other children could readily see that I used my body differently from the way they did, but neither they nor I made an issue out of it. We grew together; we played together.

Later, in junior school, I did have some problems with other students. However, it was because we were all so terribly insecure at that age. The fat girl who taunted me for not having a boyfriend did not have one herself. By high school, things ebbed back to normal.

At the end of my sophomore year, my father changed jobs and we moved to Winchester, Massachusetts. I finished high school there and applied to college.

If I may jump ahead for a moment, one unfortunate by-product of our move was that it put us close to Boston, the medical capital of the world... What happened was that everyone to whom my mother spoke urged her to take me to a particular doctor at a particular hospital. So she did.

A DISASTROUS OPERATION

After having experienced only the gentle and human approach of Dr Keats and his Easter Seal therapists, going to that hospital was like stepping into the twilight zone. Dr P., the high-powered young orthopaedist whom I saw, had little interest in me as a person. As he said, he was 'a leg doctor and not a shrink'. Although he thought I was a hopeless case, since neurological damage is neurological damage, he also took the paradoxical view that my main goal in life should be to improve my condition. It took him a while to do so, but he finally convinced my parents that it was imperative that he operate on me.

The idea of surgery made me ill, but I grew tired of fighting my parents and Dr P., who, I was told, was a nationally known expert, and at last I agreed to an operation. Dr P. severed the adductor muscle in my right leg the summer between my freshman and sophomore years at Wellesley. Before surgery, the appearance of my walk was strange and my right leg, in particular, turned in. My walk was fairly steady, though, and with a little exertion I could, when necessary, manage a close to normal clip. Sometimes I went walking for the joy of it. I had never been in hospital before. I had never experienced any prolonged discomfort ...

Nothing good came from the muscle severing, not physically or emotionally. The aim of the surgery had been to have my right leg turned out, but all the surgery did was to weaken my leg. Since the operation, my gait has been an unbalanced stagger in slow motion. My anger at what was done to me essentially against my will has never lessened.

My parents' assumption that Dr P. was an expert in physical rehabilitation turned out to be tragically inaccurate.

ON TO COLLEGE LIFE

But back to my academic life. I had finished high school in a blaze of glory... to Wellesley College.

The only accommodation Wellesley made for me was that I was allowed to type my exams. I didn't get extra time to do them, though. I did not want it. After my surgery, it took me longer to walk from place to place on campus, but I managed. There was nothing else to do but manage. Like everyone else, I formed permanent friendships with several women at Wellesley, had casual friendships with many others, and did not get along with a few. I was close to two teachers. I was a good student, but not an excellent one, a Wellesley College Scholar, not a Durant Scholar. In many important ways, my experience at Wellesley was quite typical.

The most serious drawback of Wellesley for me was that it was a women's school. I have always had my best shot at relationships (platonic or otherwise) with men if we can get to know each other in everyday situations. Most of my friends met men at mixed parties. However, since success at mixers depends so much on the first impression one makes physically, such parties were not a viable way for me to meet men. I spent four years without any male companionship and I wasn't the better for it. That is why, if I had to do it over again, I'd go to a co-ed school.

EARNING A LAW DEGREE

I became a senior in 1974, at the height of the women's movement. The emphasis was on careers with a capital 'C' and half my friends were applying to law school. I decided I might as well apply, too... That year Harvard Law School accepted ten women from Wellesley. I was among them.

Since 1977, after Harvard, I have been employed an an attorney in Hartford, Connecticut. I specialise in state regulation of automobile and homeowners' insurance, contract drafting, and copyrights. My job is not thrilling, but it is a good job and I try to take a conscientious attitude towards it.

During my first years in the Hartford area, I felt at sea in a strange, out-of-the-way place. Slowly, I have made friends and forged connections here. Hartford is home for me now, at least for the time being.

Things do not always go well. Sometimes I go out with men, but for long stretches there may be no one. I have bouts of depression. Increasingly, I am angry when people make assumptions about me solely because of my gait or my speech, and this happens daily. Yet the fact remains, I am an independent adult woman, which is pretty much what I always wanted to be.

One of the good things that has happened to me over the past few years has been my coming to better terms with my physical self. For a long time after my ill-fated surgery, I felt extremely alienated from my body. Now I realise that there is so much about my body that is right. I have splendid general health and I need a bare seven hours of sleep a night to function well. With one exception, I have not consulted a doctor in reference to my disability in the last ten years. Athetosis presents practical problems, not medical problems. However, I have taken yoga and currently I have a general exercise programme. The increase in my self-esteem about my physical self has had side effects. I used to buy clothes for work at discount stores – no polyester shift was too cheap for me. Now I buy many of my clothes at specialty shops.

A few weeks ago when I was having lunch at a coffee shop, I spilled some ketchup. A woman at a table near mine shook her grey head sadly. I remained silent, but I wanted to tell her that she shouldn't be so concerned. For who among us has not spilled ketchup? Only those who do not indulge in ketchup. ●

EMPLOYMENT – THE STRUGGLE CONTINUES □

There is often a far-reaching – and mistaken – assumption that women who are disabled do not need to work, that their financial security will be provided by their families and that their main role will be at home because their capacity to do much else is limited. In addition, society also assumes the disabled woman should not marry.

Labour market policies ignore the fact that many women are responsible for the financial security of their families: one-third of all heads of households are women, and many more families are supported by women in the absence of men who are working away from home, or are at war or unemployed. Disabled women can also be heads of households, either because along with the able-bodied they take on family commitments, or because disability strikes them later in life while they are fulfilling those commitments. There is evidence that onset of disability for an older woman may lead to being deserted or divorced, thus making her the head of a household and therefore in need of income for her family to survive.[15]

Furthermore, the growing self-help and 'independent living' movements are motivating women with disability toward joining the increasing number of women in the labour force. It is estimated that by the year 2000, more than 1 billion women – one-third of the world's female population – will be consistency economically active. A great proportion of these women will be working in the services sector and many in part-time jobs.

At first glance it would have seemed that part-time work might be ideal for women of different types of disability... Competition, however, is often intense for part-time jobs. As disabled workers are often viewed with suspicion in case they may be frequently ill, absent or unable to stand the pace, they are less likely to be successful landing jobs.

Moreover, in some member states (in the European Community), disabled women are even further discriminated against because if they work part-time they will lose many of their disability-related benefits yet not earn enough money to make up for these losses.[16]

But, there is good news for disabled women who are seeking paid employment in today's fast-changing, technology-dominated world of work. As society moves into the post-industrial era, rapid technological progress has already completely transformed the workplace as computer-based production processes automate manufacturing. Information-processing technology is fuelling the phenomenal growth of the services sector, in which the majority of workers are women.

Physical work is giving way to jobs that require more brains than muscles, a welcome development for physically disabled job-seekers. This could mean that many jobs previously closed to disabled people because of physical requirements may now be open to them.

> A women with disability needs to have a lot to offer to convince an employer to look beyond both her gender and her disability.

Technology is also paving the way for easier participation of disabled people in the workforce with the introduction of special aids and adaptations. Optacons, Versabraille, Braille speech printers, speech synthesisers, voice recognition, voice communication option boards in computers for direct telephony by the hearing-impaired, and brain/computer interface technology have already gone a very long way to diminish the disadvantage of the person with a disability in the world of work.

The preference for intellectual skills over physical ones, flexibility as regards place, time and pacing, and the growth in the number of sophisticated technical aids are features of the new technology that can bring many disabled people closer to the potential of a job, even a rather good job.

So much for the good news. Technology has not, however, come up with a way to change employers' negative attitudes towards women employees generally and disabled women in particular. Many resist providing the technology that would enable the worker who is disabled to enter the new marketplace as an equal; the 'employers' limited knowledge of disability, associated with prejudices and fears about the high cost of health and work benefits and insurance cost, can

definitely erase many or all chances of employment for disabled women'.[17] Employers by and large take a dim view of the legislation in many Western countries that provides for incentives for hiring disabled workers such as cash payments to provide employment aids and adaptations, subsidies to make up for loss of productivity, quotas or a requirement of policies for employing persons with disabilities.

It is interesting to note that in many instances the commitment of large commercial organisations to hiring, training and developing technology suitable for disabled people often derives from the actions of specific individuals within the company. Sometimes these may be owners or top management, but the erratic nature of these procedures underlines the haphazard nature of the readiness of some of these organisations to become involved with hiring disabled employees.[18]

A woman with disability needs to have a lot to offer if she is to compete with the non-disabled and convince an employer to look beyond her gender and her disability. This could be a difficult task indeed in the new world of work where the planning, communication skills and teamwork skills that are required presuppose a confidence and independence which the life experience of a woman with disability does little to encourage.

Centres still provide outmoded skills □ Moreover, there is a curious attitude among many rehabilitation professionals that technology is something they do not have to understand; this puts into question the theory that technology is making the placement of people with disabilities much easier. All too many vocational rehabilitation training centres are still providing disabled people with skills for jobs that are no longer needed on local labour markets. One reason given for this odd state of affairs is that the centres can

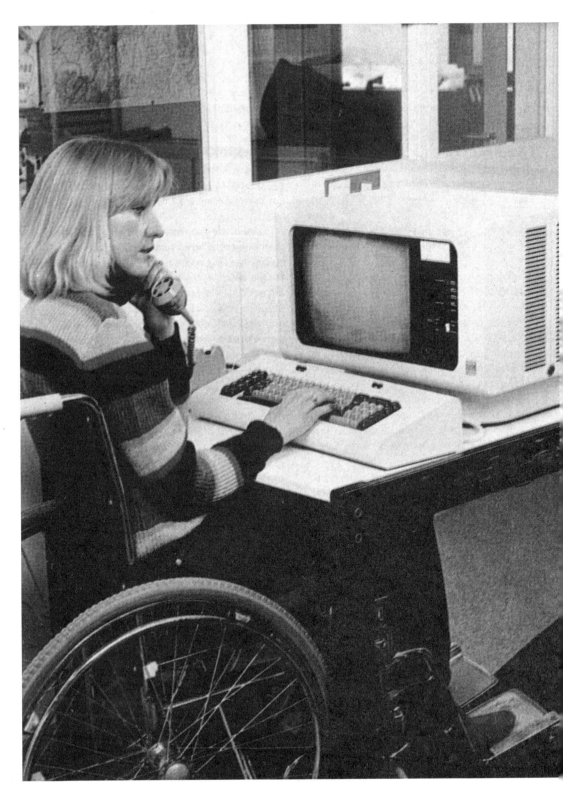

not afford to keep up with the advance of technology in the workplace! It would seem that if the centres want to be effective at all, they cannot afford not to.

At this comparatively early stage of the automated information age, experts are already warning of a polarisation of jobs into top level, decision-making posts – occupied chiefly by men – and the routine jobs (which risk further deskilling as technology continues to progress) to which the great majority of women are assigned.

Despite the growing numbers of women in the labour forces of Western countries and the progress made through vigorous feminist lobbying, the age-old view lingers stubbornly on that women are economically dependent on men.

Their work outside the home seems secondary, requiring less educational attainment, providing limited access to training, promotion and managerial positions, less job satisfaction, lower status and offering lower pay. Much more subtly, male attitudes to women and work may range from paternalism, through indifference to hostility, with the result that many women learn not to challenge, accept lower status and achievement, and develop a 'feminine' approach that is acceptable to men. Relevant literature indicates that underlying attitudes result in disabled women being offered fewer options, having lower aspirations and accepting a greater degree of dependency than their disability requires.[19]

Neutered' data □ A further problem is the absence of solid data on these subjects.

There is a lack of reliable data relating to disabled women which prevents, among other things, the identification of trends on their being among the employed and unemployed workforces. In fact, the bulk of the meager statistical data about the employment of disabled people is in general given in a 'neutered' way. That is, it is presented without making any distinction between sexes or between the different age levels, as... is normally done in the more general statistics periodically furnished by governments, concerning the employment and unemployment situation... It is self-explanatory and requires no further comment, the fact that disabled women generally do not even represent a significant entity to be taken into consideration for statistical studies, even when these studies are specifically related to disability problems.[20]

The ILO has carried out a number of studies on the situation of women with disabilities in Africa and Asia and has organised a series of meetings to improve the employment opportunities for them and their female children.

In many developing countries, mentally retarded women have been trained to look after domestic animals and help in planting and harvesting crops. Good therapy, perhaps, but hardly remunerative. Piecework at home is prevalent among women generally and provides a low return for long hours of work, sometimes with unsafe materials and under questionable conditions. The employers obtain cheap labour and the women have no legal or social security protection. Disabled women who are sometimes involved in this kind of work are even more vulnerable to exploitation.

A survey of women and disability in the Philippines revealed that only 19 per cent of disabled women were employed. Furthermore, 95 per cent of those who were employed had to settle for very low wages, earning an average of only $35.38 per month – an income that is not even one-third of the poverty threshold set by the World Bank at $130.65 for rural areas.[21]

Employment was one of the chief cate

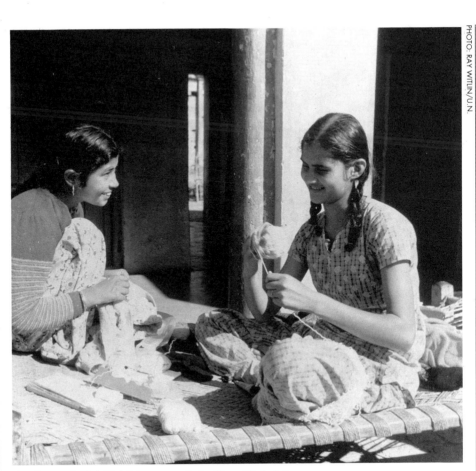

The right to work: blind girls knitting garments in the village of Ugala, India.

gories included in surveys carried out in 1987 to ascertain the needs of disabled women in Fiji, India, Japan, Pakistan, the Philippines and Thailand. The project was sponsored by the ILO. Survey findings showed that, taking the six countries as a whole, one-third of 767 disabled women respondents were working in some capacity, 30 per cent were neither working nor studying, 21 per cent were students or trainees and 15 per cent were housewives or engaged in household work.

Independence achieved through employment was the ultimate goal of the majority of the students who were questioned... Apprehension, however,

tended to dim the students' hopes for the future – apprehension that because of their disability they will not be able to perform a job satisfactorily – apprehension that in the world of work they will find the same discrimination and rejection from employers and co-workers that they experienced in school from teachers and fellow students.

Where information on the limitations imposed by disability on job opportunities and performance was provided, the respondents were unanimous in asserting that the existence of a disability was the root cause of the on-the-job difficulties they

encountered – lost job opportunities and discrimination. For some, it created barriers to communication with colleagues and for others it diminished their ability to work a full 8-hour day. Because many of the respondents had pre-employment difficulties in attending a school for the non-disabled and found that educational opportunities in special schools were limited, they could qualify for only menial jobs.

Unable to cope with these difficulties, many of the women who had full-time jobs gave them up for lower paying, part-time work or opted out of the labour force entirely.[22]

Employment is important for persons with disabilities and particularly for women with disabilities. It can provide economic security and independence and give them value and status as individuals. It helps with integration and acceptance by the non-disabled and, most important-ly, it gives life a purpose.

A SURVEY OF WOMEN WITH DISABILITIES IN NON-TRADITIONAL CAREERS
Joanne Slappo and Lynda J. Katz

A sample of 449 women with disabilities in non-traditional careers from across the USA was surveyed in order to determine: (a) what factors contributed to choice of career; (b) what factors contributed to success in career; (c) what career prob-lems were encountered; (d) what career problems were unique to them; and (e) what factors contributed to solving career problems (see 3 tables overleaf). Usable surveys received from 170 women indicat-ed that women with disabilities in non-tra-ditional careers, especially those in profes-sional occupations, were, in many respects, like their non-disabled counter-

parts. Women with disabilities in the study were predominantly white, in their mid-thirties, unmarried, considered themselves high academic achievers and reported hav-ing a great deal of personal initiative, per-sistence and assertiveness. The majority of the women were in professional, non-tra-ditional occupations, a great percentage of them working for large companies and earning salaries well above the average for working women with disabilities. High salaries, personal satisfaction, and intellec-tual and emotional stimulation were expe-rienced by the majority of women in the study. These benefits, however, appeared to be more readily available to women in professional occupations than to those in skilled or semi-skilled positions. Factors that distinguished women with disabilities from their non-disabled counterparts were the career problems experienced. The most serious obstacles to careers are reported as being the following: people's attitudes towards individuals with disabili-ties, having a disability, and being a woman with a disability. ●

ACCESS TO TRAINING AND EMPLOYMENT IN RURAL OCCUPA-TIONS AND CO-OPERATIVES*
Grace Ingham-Wright

Blind women have a right to indepen-dence and self-expression. Women and girls expect to have their own place in the environment in to which they are born and to which they have become accus-tomed. Most women have a desire to be needed and have future aspirations to be strived for.

To those who have to find their niche in

---

* Excerpts from a paper presented to the International Conference on the Situation of Blind Women, Belgrade, November 1975. Grace Ingham-Wright is Senior Community Projects Organiser, London Borough of Merton.

PROFESSIONAL NON-TRADITIONAL CAREERS – reported by 104 survey respondents

OCCUPATION	NO.	OCCUPATION	NO.
Aerospace physiologist	1	*Pharmaceutical companies*	
Air traffic control operator	1	Formulation control co-ordinator	1
Architect	1	Pharmacist	3
Attorney	11	Physician	4
Chemist	2	Physicist	1
Child psychiatrist	1	Physiologist	1
Computer marketing representative	1	Position classification specialist	1
Computer programmer/analyst	12	Research specialist	1
Computer project manager/supervisor	3	*Professors of*	
Defence contract specialist	1	Biology	1
Engineer	3	Chemistry	1
Engineer technician	2	Dentistry	1
Geologist	2	Geology	1
Industrial designer	1	History	1
Laboratory technician	1	Medical	6
Legislative specialist	2	Microbiology	1
Manager constituent relations	1	Psychiatry	1
Marketing and programme director	1	Rehabilitation	3
Maths co-ordinator	1	Sociology	1
Medical researcher	2	Promotions assistant	1
Microbiologist	4	Public affairs assistant	1
Minister	4	Rehabilitation counsellor	1
Musician	1	Science lecturer and consultant	1
Nuclear inspector	1	Scientist	3
Operations research analyst	1	Self-employed (owner of company)	2
Orthodontist	1	Statistician	2
Maintenance worker	1	Store manager	1
		Union organiser	1

SKILLED/SEMI-SKILLED NON-TRADITIONAL CAREERS – reported by 16 survey respondents

OCCUPATION	NO.	OCCUPATION	NO.
Bander	1	Oil burner tester	1
Cleaner and inspector	1	Plastics operator	1
Dismantler	1	Postal carrier	1
Drafter	2	Security officer	1
Escort driver	1	Shipping/receiving clerk	2
Forklift Operator	1	Tool and die maker	1
Maintenance worker	1	Trainer (manufacturing)	1

DEMOGRAPHIC DATA ON SURVEY RESPONDENTS IN NON-TRADITIONAL CAREERS

	PROFESSIONALS		SKILLED/SEMI-SKILLED		TOTAL	
	No.	%	No.	%	No.	%
Marital status						
Never married	53	51.0	6	37.5	59	49.2
Married	34	32.7	1	6.3	35	29.2
Widowed	2	1.9	1	6.3	3	2.5
Separated	2	1.9	3	18.8	5	4.2
Divorced	12	11.5	3	18.8	15	12.5
N/A	1	1.0	2	12.5	3	2.5
Children						
None	77	74.0	7	43.8	84	70.0
Under 5 years	8	7.7			8	6.7
6–11 years	5	4.8	3	18.8	8	6.7
12–17 years	4	3.8	5	31.3	9	7.5
18+ years	14	13.6	4	25.0	18	14.9
Racial status						
White	97	93.3	13	81.3	110	91.7
Black	2	1.9	-	-	2	1.7
American Indian	-	-	1	6.3	1	0.8
Hispanic	1	1.0	-	-	1	0.8
Other	2	1.9	-	-	2	1.7
N/A	2	1.9	2	12.5	4	3.3
Onset of disability						
Birth	28	26.9	6	37.5	34	28.3
1–20 years	56	53.8	2	12.5	58	48.3
21–52 years	20	19.0	8	50.0	28	23.3

Note: *The average ages for the professional, skilled/semi-skilled, and total categories represented above were 38.6, 35.7, and 36.9 years respectively.*

the rural areas of any country, blindness is an obstacle. In developing countries, education is almost impossible and marriage is often out of the question. When blindness occurs after marriage, the effect on the family is disruptive, with the blind wife being often misunderstood and sometimes deserted by her husband. Her children are cared for by relatives and, because of over-anxiety, the blind wife is left in a place of safety with no mental or physical outlet.

When young blind girls become pregnant they rarely have the joy of bringing up their children; the babies are taken away by older women in the family. Very few men will consider themselves as the prospective husband of such a person and it appears that there is no future for her.

Rural village women and girls can be assisted to become useful members of society whether born blind or if they suffer loss of sight later in life.

When planning a rehabilitation project with a view to future employment in rural occupations, it is necessary to have a close, sympathetic understanding of the area in which the work is to be undertaken. A start must be made from the grass-roots if lasting progress is to take place...

Training of a basic and simple nature in the home of the person chosen can achieve spectacular results, especially when the young woman is newly blind but has already received from the family her initial training as a prospective bride or young wife. Most newly blind women rehabilitate themselves within the confines of their own homes. Necessity dictates that they must do so. After initial blunders they rapidly become once more adept within a household that they themselves have arranged and planned. It is often more necessary to educate the immediate family to remember that there is a place for everything, and everything must be in its place.

After basic household training in cleaning, cooking and budgeting comes childcare. No more must she lose her babies to others. They are an insurance for the future as well as a present joy to the proud young mother... Useful occupations, which are also gainful monetarily, are the final parts of a successful training project. These must be suited to the area, as there is nothing more ludicrous than training a blind person in a skill which is not saleable within the community or at an easily accessible market. Any skills taught must be to a very high standard, so that the end product is much prized, sought after and paid for...

In West Africa the most popular and favourite method of arousing a young blind woman out of apathy proved to be a dance in the compound... To the surprise and indeed often the amazement of her family she would tentatively join in after some initial encouragement from the trainers. It was not long before she was dancing to the well-known songs sung from childhood. The social attitude of the family begins its slow change from then on.

It is generally found that the blind young woman has had skills taught to her in the past, and only requires encouragement to start again... The child born blind is not so lucky unless she has a very strong character and is allowed to roam freely around the village. Work with this type of woman is more complex and requires much more patience and understanding. Usually good results come from associating the one born blind with a successful blind housewife, for no one can better teach a blind person than a person who is blind herself...

The co-operative movement is a natural end result, whether by a group of blind women, or by a mixed group, working together in the village.

Somewhere within the co-operative movement the blind woman can hold her

Miss Joyce Bulera (right), manager of the sheltered workshop at Masaka in Souther Uganda, helps a disabled woman hand-print cotton cloth. Twenty severely handicapped people have found employment here.

47

own when given the chance to prove her-self. A co-operative of women in an African village employed two blind women who had been trained to care for their children whilst they went to market. Another group organised themselves into a village co-operative including the trained blind women, who quickly found they could direct the others into more profitable channels. Business boomed and the status of the women improved until they were considered as the most highly respected women in the village. One mar-ried the local schoolmaster and the other sits in the local market directing opera-tions.

To enable the blind worker to be really productive and financially helpful to her family, a rural co-operative, organised so that the most skilled person takes the goods or produce to sell in the market whilst the workers remain busily occupied in their homes, is a sound practice. This follows the pattern used by the sighted market women throughout West Africa...

The blind young woman must have a sense of achievement, but no complacen-cy. She should be able to accept her place in life as a right, but must understand that an effort must be made to keep that posi-tion. It is her own life, her own effort and her own achievement...

FIGHTING PREJUDICE WITH SKILLS
Existing evidence indicates that the best way to combat prejudice against the dis-abled, men or women, is to provide the disabled persons with skills and/or income-generating activities that help to restore the productive value of people with disabilities in the eyes of the non-disabled and remove them from the category of helpless, dependent people who can only be a burden to others and objects of pity. ●

WOMEN IN REHABILITATION – WHY AND WHY NOT? *
Eunice Fiorito and Jim Doherty

...The male bias which pervades rehabilita-tion and vocational training schemes for the disabled is also clearly reflected in male domination of decision-making in rehabilitation organisations. For women who choose rehabilitation as a professional field, somewhere along the line they are usually made abruptly conscious of this situation once they reach a certain level in the hierarchy. Following are excerpts of an article co-authored by a female vet-eran of the battle of the sexes as it is waged in government rehabilitation agen-cies – she tells it like it is... Regrettably, extensive research regarding women in the rehabilitation field does not yet exist. Therefore, the statements and opinions expressed here are based on personal experience and countless discussions with female colleagues. The situations described are real. They outline clearly the position of women in this profession but, admittedly, do not document it. The entire system would benefit from a comprehensive sur-vey that would produce reliable statistics on the number of women in the field, what levels of responsibility they occupy, how professional advancement varies for women and men and how professional degrees are distributed between the sexes. In addition, researchers should examine the feelings and attitudes of women, ask-ing such questions as why did they choose rehabilitation work? what were their expectations? how have these dreams been altered and by what circumstances? how were the women counselled in high school

* Extracts from Eunice Fiorito and Jim Doherty, 'Women in rehabilitation – why and why not?', *Rehabilitation World*, winter 1983–84. Eunice Fiorito is Acting Director of the Division of Special Projects, Rehabilitation Service Administration, US Department of Education. Jim Doherty is a freelance writer.

and college? what do they view as their accomplishments and disappointments in their work? how do they relate to male co-workers and superiors? and how do they cope with a system which is directed by men but depends for its effectiveness on great numbers of women.

MANY START AS VOLUNTEERS

The tradition of directing women into the helping professions is not based solely on fanciful notions. Women do seem to have an instinctive desire to help, to nurture and care for people. Many have said they chose rehabilitation work for this reason. Others, who entered higher education with no clearly defined career decision, say they were steered, at least indirectly, toward the field by teachers and advisors who stressed the helping aspect of the job. A great many women now employed in various phases of rehabilitation work report that their first exposure to the field came through volunteer activity. Not surprisingly, the vast majority of rehabilitation volunteers are women. Their value and influence will be considered later.

Discussions with female colleagues have produced a pattern of professional progress that occurs too often to be called coincidental. A woman is hired as a counsellor. Her case assignments indicate a belief in her capability. She is praised by her superiors for 'being so good with people'. Naturally, she is pleased to be considered a success. At this point, she does not understand that this praise might one day work against her potential advancement.

FIGURES BEAR OUT MALE DOMINATION

The hidden barrier takes the form of statements such as, 'We would hate to take you away from the clients. You work so well and have such great rapport with

them.' As a result, women tend to be concentrated in low- and mid-level positions. Jacqueline Packer has presented graphic evidence of this. In an article in the *Journal of Visual Impairment and Blindness*, she outlines the characteristics of rehabilitation professionals who responded to a detailed survey she conducted. When asked for their occupational title, 56 per cent of the men and a like number of women wrote 'vocational rehabilitation counsellor'. However, at the level of administrator/supervisor/manager, 34 per cent of the men but only 22 per cent of the women could claim the title. Even more dramatic figures appeared in the section on persons supervised: 33 per cent of the men and 40 per cent of the women responding were in charge of groups of one to four persons. When the group was somewhat larger, five to eight employees, 20 per cent of the men and 60 per cent of the women were classified as supervisors. But above that level, all administrative power was in male hands: 47 per cent of the men were responsible for staffs larger than eight.

Even some men might agree that these figures support the charge of 'male domination'. But they would probably also claim that women are gradually moving into more managerial positions. However, what they call 'managerial' is really 'supervisory'. From these somewhat higher positions, women continue to work primarily with people, while the male managers continue to design programmes and promulgate policies.

> '...mid-level male staffers are recognized as experts in senior staff meetings while women are expected to serve coffee and take notes'.

To some extent, and certainly inadvertently, female volunteers have helped to shape the pattern outlined above.

49

Volunteers perform a variety of essential services that make rehabilitation productive both for clients and agency staffs, all for the best of reasons and no pay. Some male administrators use this dedication to helping as the basis for reasoning that under-rewards the contributions of female staff members and keeps them in direct-service positions. In some agencies, this kind of thinking shows itself all too obviously in work assignments and meeting participation. Women report instances in which mid-level male staff are recognised as experts in senior staff meetings, while women are expected to serve coffee and take minutes...

The rehabilitation system is suffering because women do not share programme direction and leadership. If it is valid to say that women are especially effective in working with people, then the system loses a great deal when the ability is confined to lower levels. Insights gained through day-to-day dealings with clients could bring important information to planning sessions. By keeping the inner sanctum doors open to men only, agencies are depriving themselves and those they serve of a vital resource.

Thus far, the discussion of women in rehabilitation has been rather one-sided. That is not entirely fair. Tradition and the 'old boy network' are indeed the principal forces restricting the upward mobility of women in the field, but we women are also to blame. Like other minorities, we have usually accepted our assigned status becuase 'it's better than nothing' – which is the constantly frightening alternative. Some of us even deny the fact of discrimination because we don't want to admit to an unequal position.

The field of rehabilitation – counselling, planning and administration – is full of opportunity for creative, positive action on behalf of individuals and the system itself. Women have demonstrated superior performance in every job category that is equally open to us. We can be justly proud of the work we have done. We must now be more assertive in seeking just reward for our accomplishments. ●

1 Dr Salma Maqbool, 'Development of leadership of women with disabilities', Leadership Training Seminar, Bangkok, Thailand, September 1988.
2 *Report of the Workshop on the Development of Policies and Programmes for Disabled Women and Female Disabled Children in the Southern African Region.* The workshop was organised by the ILO and funded by the Norwegian International Development Agency and the Arab Gulf Fund, and held in Harare, Zimbabwe, in September 1985.
3 Dr Einar Helander, The WHO Program for Community-based Rehabilitation in International Rehabilitation Review, December 1988.
4 Ibid.
5 Mary Croxen John, 'Vocational rehabilitation of disabled women in the European Community', sponsored by the Commission of the European Community Bureau for Action in Favour of Disabled People, November 1988.
6 Sheila Stace, *Vocational Rehabilitation for Women with Disabilities,* ILO, Geneva, 1986.
7 *Report of the Workshop on the Development of Policies and Programmes for Disabled Women and Female Disabled Children in the Southern African Regions* ILO, 1985.
8 Ibid.
9 Susan R. Hammerman, 'Women and disability', Rehabilitation International Conference on Women with Disabilities, New York, February 1986.
10 Dr Valerie Ellien, 'Women and disability: an international perspective', *Rehabilitation World,* winter 1984.
11 Ibid.
12 Dr Y. Kojima, 'Strategies to improve socio-vocational integration of disabled women in Japan', from research sponsored by the International Labour Office, Tokyo, 1988.
13 *Beacon* (the newsletter of the Divine Light Trust for the Blind), October 1988.
14 *International Rehabilitation Review,* December 1985.
15 Shiela Stace, *Vocational Rehabilitation for Women with Disabilities,* ILO, Geneva, 1986.
16 Mary Croxen John, *The Vocational Rehabilitiation for Disabled Women in the European Community* November 1988.
17 Dr Denise G. Tate, 'Women and disability: a review of problems and facts', *Proceedings of World Congress of Rehabilitation International,* Lisbon, 1984.
18 John Moses 'Preparing for the brave new workplace: the impact of new technology on the employment of people with disabilities', *International Rehabilitation Review,* December 1988, pp. 7–9.
19 Shiela Stace, *Vocational Rehabilitation for Women with Disabilities,* ILO, Geneva, 1986.
20 Dra Teresa Selli Serra, 'The impact of disability on women', *Proceedings of the 15th World Congress of Rehabilitation International,* Lisbon, 1984.

21 Ruby Gonzales, 'Employment: women with disabilities', conference papers, n.d.

22 'Dispelling the shadows of neglect: a survey on women with disabilities in six Asian and Pacific countries', ILO, 1989.

4 THE HUMAN RIGHTS OF DISABLED WOMEN

In an era marked by highly visible opposition to the infringement of human rights, disabled women are systematically denied the most human of rights – the right to love, the right to marriage, the right to motherhood, the right to personal fulfilment. While disabled men are more likely to marry, to enjoy the blessings of family life, in some societies it is considered somehow shocking that a disabled woman should marry, and families are usually the most vehement in discouraging any aspirations disabled women may have to fulfil a woman's destiny.

THE ABLE-BODIED often treat women who have disabilities as asexual. Nothing could be further from the truth, but as a result of such attitudes, disabled women often flee into social isolation.

THE IMPORTANCE OF SEXUALITY □

The sexuality of a woman with a handicap is just as much a part of her identity as it is for a non-disabled woman.

Women with a disability must contend with the media's image of the perfect woman complete with the perfect body, the myth of the oversexed or asexual disabled woman, and the feminine mystique which is defined by a traditional, heterosexual marriage complete with children and possibly a job. Sexuality of women with mental handicaps has consequently been either ignored or

denied. The importance of sexuality to the well-being of all women needs to be recognised.[1]

Disabled women are increasingly outspoken on the once-taboo subject of their sexuality.

All too often, society at large fails to recognise the universality of this fundamental truth and sees disabled people as not entitled to love, helping to impose barriers and inhibitions and encouraging the repression of their sexuality. Thus, disabled people have not only their own difficulties to overcome but also the prejudices and fears of so-called 'normal' people often acting out their own inadequacies.

Anxious parents, who have devotedly cared for their handicapped child through its early years, are often bewildered when it comes to coping with the difficulties of adolescence. They play it safe and try to protect their child from ideas and aspirations which they feel can never be fulfilled, and feel threatened and worried by overt signs of sexuality.

All adolescents are likely to experience emotional turmoil; how much more difficult for the handicapped youngsters whose rebellious and sexual inclinations can be more effectively discouraged. Striving for independence and sexual development are not easily reconciled with the necessity of accepting care.

It requires a considerable step for parents to accept that sex education plays a vital part in development, and that exposure to risks and disappointments plays a normal part in the growth of the individual as much for a disabled as for an able-bodied child. It is necessary to 'see beyond the wheelchair', to understand the capacity for sexual expression of people as they are, to recognise that imperfections and

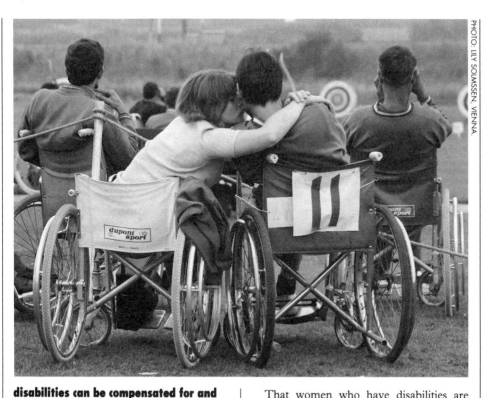

disabilities can be compensated for and the precious prize of sexual fulfilment achieved against the odds.'
For many disabled people, problems of disability are compounded by loneliness. Such isolation quickly reinforces any sexual inadequacy already felt. What is needed is the opportunity for disabled people to meet potential partners in an encouraging atmosphere. In the UK, the Outsiders Club is pioneering a new approach to social contact. Anther concerned organisation is Sexual and Personal Relationships of Disabled People (SPOD). This enterprising body provides an educational and advisory service to help disabled people overcome sexual and personal problems. Internationally, the International Forum for Sexuality and Disability seeks to pursue initiatives for progress in the enlightenment and understanding of the needs of disabled people.[2]

That women who have disabilities are increasingly outspoken on the once taboo subject of their sexuality was evident during a two-day conference held in Melbourne, Australia in June 1988 on Sexuality and Women with Disabilities. Discussions covered coming to terms with sexuality, rights as a sexual person, establishing, working within and maintaining relationships, sexual values and sexual options and sexuality for women in residential and institutional care. One issue identified by participants at the conference, particularly of those living in isolated areas, was the desire to be able to discuss sexuality with their peers in small group settings.

Then there is the dark side to sexuality for women with disability: they are fair game for the aggressions of others and they are helpless victims more often than society is aware.

Men who want dependent women search you out. You have to be careful to assess their motives in wanting a personal relationship with you. We are often questioned about our sexuality, having to fight all the misinformation about women's sexuality in general and, additionally, ignorance about disabled people's sexual abilities.[3]

The shocking incidence of violence against disabled women was brought forcibly to the attention of the March 1987 workshop of the Coalition of Provincial Organisations of the Handicapped in Winnipeg, Canada, in a paper by Cathy McPherson. She minces no words...

VIOLENCE AS IT AFFECTS DISABLED WOMEN: A VIEW FROM CANADA*
Cathy McPherson

I became aware of violence and women with disabilities when a series of rapes and murders took place one summer in Toronto, spreading a climate of fear among able-bodied women in our city.

The disabled women I know complained that the special concerns of women with disabilities were not even being considered, that physically disabled women were being raped and assaulted while waiting for parallel transportation to pick them up in darkly lit areas, or by cab drivers. Women with psychiatric disabilities were being assaulted in boarding houses with poor security and in institutions themselves, yet their word held little credibility.

Many of the bag ladies and street people with psychiatric problems had been so traumatized by the sexual abuse they had received as children and the violent assaults on the street they wouldn't associate with men at drop-in centres. Deaf women and developmentally disabled women were particularly angry at being perceived as being 'dumb' and available for sex.

PUBLIC REACTION

The women at our rape crisis centre confirmed my suspicions that there seemed to be a public perception of either horror that such an unthinkable thing could happen to someone so vulnerable and unable to protect herself; disbelief that anyone would want to have sex with a disabled woman; or, conversely, the attitude that the victim should be glad she got 'lucky' because she probably never would get the opportunity to have sex again.

My awareness of the problem came closer to home when I received a call one day informing me that a disabled member of the local group of which I was a member was in a home for battered women.

Her husband was also involved in the group and the subject became so emotionally charged that it became necessary for the women in our group to close our discussions to men. Despite the obvious need for the women to form a group of their own where women could talk in a safe and confidential atmosphere about their problems and generally about the concerns of women with disabilities without fear of intimidation, the men in our little organization had a hard time accepting this, even though we encouraged them to get their own discussion group going and gave them the names of men who were already holding discussion groups of this kind.

Like any other self-help group, our women's group was simply an opportunity to give each other encouragement and work on accessibility to women's facilities. Interestingly, some time later, I received a call from a young deaf woman who was living at home, and wanted to break out of

---

* Reprinted from Proceedings of Coalition of Provincial Organisations of the Handicapped in Winnipeg (COPOH) Workshop on Disabled Women's Issues, March 1987.

an incestuous relationship with her father by seeing a counsellor. We had a really tough time arranging for a sign language interpreter for a therapist working in this area and finding a way to get someone, apart from the woman herself, to pay for this service.

I think these last examples illustrate what we already know in our organization – that the disabled community has the same social problems as the community at large – and violence against women is one of them. If able-bodied men and women are caught up in abusive situations, then it stands to reason that disabled men and women will experience the same problems.

But where a non-disabled woman has a difficult time leaving a man who is abusing her, disabled women have an even harder time. Disabled women may have little confidence in themselves because they have been told by society that they are not attractive. As I indicated earlier, they are often encouraged by well-intentioned professionals to stay in an abusive relationship because they are told they won't get anything better.

And then there's the problem of accessibility. Even if a woman with a disability wants to get out, she may not be able to because there is little or no accessible housing available. If she has children she runs the very real risk of losing custody of her children if she leaves, particularly if her partner is non-disabled.

When I wrote an article on this some time ago, one individual angrily suggested that by talking about this openly I was scaring disabled women from going out in the community.

Certainly, rape and assault happen when people venture from their homes, and they happen more often to women than men. But the idea, I think, is to street-proof people to make sure they don't take unnecessary risks rather than encouraging self-imposed curfews on women.

Second, it is important to note that most rape, incest and sexual assault happen between women and the people who are most familiar to them – family members and friends of the family or neighbours. In the case of a woman with a disability, this often can include their attendants, institutional staff and sometimes even their doctors or therapists.

I think our organization has to take a strong stand about this and make it clear to society that it does not condone such behaviour against women and that facilities for victims of violence must be made accessible as soon as possible – as well as facilities that offer counselling services to both parties involved in the violence. ●

THE RIGHT TO MARRIAGE AND CHILDREN □ Women who are disabled have greater difficulties finding a spouse than non-disabled women or disabled men. Exceptions to this rule are the mentally retarded. While men may be more willing to marry a mentally retarded woman – especially if she is beautiful – women are more likely to refuse marriage with a mentally retarded partner.

In developing countries where, in many societies, arranged marriages are still customary, disabled women are at a great disadvantage. They also have difficulties finding a spouse because much physical labour is expected from wives in these countries – except at the highest echelons of society. Another contributing factor is the widespread fear that the presence of a disabled person in a household may bring misfortune. If a woman becomes disabled after marriage, there is a strong likelihood that her husband will leave her.

Being deserted by an unsympathetic husband would seem a preferable fate to that of a woman in India who had become disabled after marriage and whose husband had married a second wife. She told

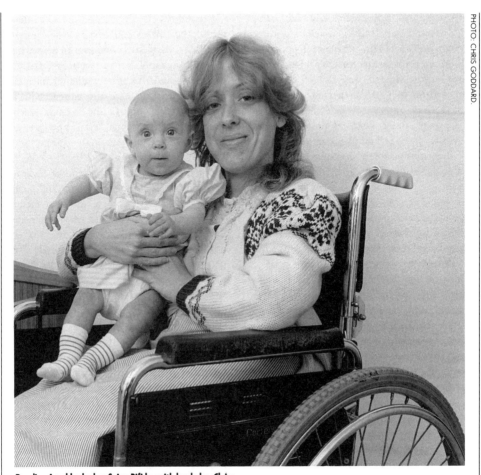

PHOTO: CHRIS GODDARD.

Rosaline Arnold who has Spina Bifida, with her baby, Claire.

a community group for the disabled that she was beaten and denied food both by her husband and his new wife. When members of the group offered to intervene, the woman would not hear of it. 'A husband is a husband,' she said, 'whether he treats me well or ill. I cannot do any harm to him.'⁴

An important issue for disabled women who do marry is the right to bear children. Here, modern science and ancient taboos go hand-in-hand to raise obstacles to the possibility of motherhood for women with disability.

Many disabled women have been counselled by medical professionals not to have children. They are told the child would suffer and that they as parents wouldn't be able to cope with emergencies. Even now, physically disabled as well as mentally disabled women run the risk of involuntary sterilisation, usually carried out in conjunction with some other operation. The medical profession gets little training about disability, yet because it is an authoritarian profession, doctors are hesitant to admit ignorance and decisions are made often on invalid premises.⁵

There is no reason why a woman who is disabled cannot have a healthy child. Few disabilities are hereditary. But decisions regarding pregnancy are often made on the basis of fear and not on well-founded information. Pregnancies of disabled women are in most cases no more difficult than those of the non-disabled. It is essential, however, to be well-informed and supervised.

Neither is a physical handicap necessarily a handicap to being a parent, which is more than just a question of physical tasks. It involves providing security and love as well as guiding the child into responsible adulthood. Certainly a disabled mother may have difficulty in carrying, bathing or feeding a child. She may have difficulty in sharing sports or play activities. But there is no indication that children of disabled mothers have a higher accident rate than those whose mothers are not disabled.

Having a disabled mother may give a child an early sense of responsibility and independence. Because of her difficulties in mobility, a disabled mother can give more attention to her children – she has more time to read to them, to help them with school work. Children are adaptable and generally can accept the disability of a parent. Unless there are extremely pressing reasons, children should not be separated from their disabled mothers. Rather, the mothers should be offered help, for example to perform certain functions of childcare.

The disabled woman and mother has to be granted all kinds of help in order to enable her to preserve her independence in the responsibility for housework and above all for the care and education of her children. This requires also a narrow network of encouraging mobile social services and the establishment of local agencies for treatment and advisory services.

Mothers with a disability have anecdotally reported services such as handibus access for delivering children to daycare as an area of service denial. There is a lack of technological aids and support services and little funding for work in this area. Mothers with handicaps, and their needs, have been ignored at least partially because there is a denial that they have a right to a family life like all other women.[6]

There is no reason that a disabled woman cannot give birth to a healthy child, but it is essential to be well-informed and supervised.

A young disabled woman who refused to be denied that right has written an informative account of how she succeeded. It has the ring of authenticity that is understandably lacking in even the best-documented papers written by experts. And a contribution for this book was requested from a young disabled Chinese woman along the lines of a 'disability and me' approach. The fact that her response was devoted solely to 'my love story' is a poignant indication of the longing that dominates the personal life of a woman who is disabled. Slightly condensed versions of the stories of these two women follow. ●

MY LOVE STORY

Zhang Li

This is my true story, a heartbreaking story. I am a seriously handicapped person, but I am a woman all the same, a woman made of flesh and blood, with feelings and love of my own. From the bottom of my heart I do love a man, no matter how bitter it feels.

He was leaving now, dragging heavy feet toward the door, his eyes brimming with tears, filled with unspeakable sorrow. As he was turning the knob, he looked back

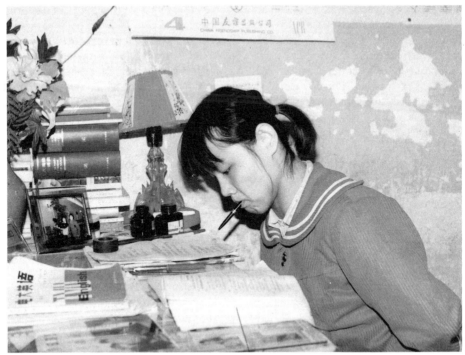

Zhang Li, Beijing Children's Welfare Institution, 1988.

silently, his gaze resting on me for a long while. Then he said in a dreadful voice, 'Lili, please wait for me!' Tears were running down his cheeks, and he dashed out.

The door closed on my ward room with an agonizing click which made my blood run cold. I threw myself on my bed and burst into tears, sobbing frantically, and my pillow and blanket were soaked with tears. Off you are now, Ting, and once more we'll have to live far away from each other, but when shall we meet again? When will it be the next time I'll be nestling against your chest?

I was lying there, crying, whispering his name again and again, but he was with me no more to give the answer. I do not know how much time elapsed until the young nurse came and brought me my dinner. 'Have your meal, Lili, and stop crying, for the good of your health!' she said, wiping my tears away with a towel. She was hold-

ing a bowl of delicious vermicelli soup with eggs and was going to feed me, but staring at it, I had no appetite at all, for my heart was aching as if torn to pieces... It was getting dark, all was quiet around, and I was sitting dazed, under the dim light of the desk lamp. I opened my diary. My eye fell at first on his picture. 'Ting, my beloved.' I pressed the picture on my cheeks and on my lips...

I did not notice when the tabby cat leapt in and came to me, looking up and mewing at me, licking my face. The clever thing seemed to be aware that I was weeping my eyes out, and it had come to console me. I caught it in my lap. 'You pussycat, only you understand me!' Bitter tears reminded me how I made his acquaintance several years earlier. It was four years ago.

In the second half of 1984, in the Beijing Welfare Hospital for Children, an extraordinarily handicapped girl made herself known. She was badly crippled and had been bedridden for years, surviving only thanks to daily medication. But her will-power finally got the better of her disability. In her bed, she plunged herself into self-studies. Holding her pen with her teeth, she started writing and became the authoress of quite a few short stories and stirring poems... Zhang Li was her name.

Soon my name appeared in the newspapers and magazines. Several publishers had my self-taught experience printed with spectacular headlines: 'The Young Authoress Wrote With Her Mouth', 'A Second Life', 'She Stubbornly Survived', etc. They gave a faithful and stirring report of my fight against disability, telling how I became a self-taught writer by sheer perseverance, managing to hold my pen with my mouth...

Those inspiring comments greatly moved the public. As soon as my deeds had been reported in the press, I received a flow of letters from readers. Those friends highly appreciated and meant to follow the example I had set for them. I also received many love letters from male admirers who boldly told me about their feelings. Among them were healthy and sound young men who sent me their pictures; on the prints, they all looked bright and handsome and virile. But more of them appeared to be physically handicapped boyfriends. I was amazed and I wondered how people could care for a cripple like me.

Skimming through these love letters, I noticed one with a couple of butterflies printed on it. It was the first letter I ever read of his. As I unfolded it, a big red maple leaf slipped out. I picked it up and read these two lines in a firm handwriting: 'Red like the fire burning in my heart are maple leaves, please accept this one.' I took the letter:

Lili, Forgive me for taking the liberty to write you this letter. At this very moment, I can hardly contain my emotion and my pen is trembling, and yet I do not know what to write on this sheet of paper in front of me.

My heart leapt at my first glance over today's newspapers, when those stirring headlines caught my attention. I was so impatient to know what it was all about, and I read them several times at a stretch. When I was through, my face was bathed in tears.

You are a marvellous girl. Ruthless destiny made you handicapped, and remaining a bedridden invalid is an endless torture. But, you stubborn girl, you overcame all that. You not only survived, but you achieved what normal people would never have been able to do.

My heart is pounding, my blood is boiling, and your name is jingling in my ears and your fine figure engraved in my heart... Today and today only do I realize that I have finally found the love of my life.

As I came to these words, I felt myself blushing to the roots of my hair. This fearless suitor had so much to say, and from his letter I learned he was crippled in the lower limbs, and had to walk on crutches. As to the cause of his being crippled, he did not mention a single word. He has always been rather reluctant to speak about himself. One more thing I learned about him is that he was also studying and writing, just like me...

I was quite unable to calm down after having read his letter, and I had been holding it for a long while. At the same time, this man aroused my curiosity: why didn't he tell me the story of his disability? This led me to fancy answering him.

That evening, I dragged myself along near the lamp to write him. In a short letter, I thanked him for his sincere feelings and I expressed the wish to make friends with him. Out of some sense of modesty, I did not think fit, being a girl, to give any response to his advances. Moreover, I was aware of my own serious invalidity. In my condition, how could I expect that love would come as a godsend to me? A few days later, I received another letter from him, with the same two butterflies on the envelope.

Dear Lili, It was surely with the blessing of God that I received your reply. Our coming to know each other must have been arranged by Heaven. I am clasping your letter tight to my chest and kissing it unbelievingly, as though you were facing me with your beautiful eyes shining with tenderness...

It was the will of Heaven, I said to myself. I read on to the end, and a picture fell from the envelope. On the print, he looked rather ordinary, a square face with eyes that were not very big but seemed to be filled with sadness. He looked about forty, but in fact he was only thirty-one at that time. I turned the photo over and on the back of it was written, 'Lonely I have been every day, but fortunately I met a bosom friend today!'

Since that time, letters decorated with a couple of butterflies have been flowing to me like snowflakes. Each one was very, very long, as he was eager to tell me everything about himself. He went on saying in his letter, 'Lili, your tenderness warmed up my frozen heart and I cannot wait any more, I am longing to see you, to be with you...'

I joyfully agreed, I accepted love from a man I never met. I picked out the best photograph I could find of me in the album and I wrote on the back, 'I agree, my darling. Let your love warm my heart forever!'

He came and I met him for the first time. I had received a telegram letting me know about his coming to Beijing. The third morning after I received his telegram, there was a knock at the door. I choked with emotion and tried to disguise my lack of composure before I answered,

'Please come in!'

The door opened and he was standing there in the doorway, soberly dressed, holding a crutch, a big travelling bag slung across his shoulder. He looked tired after a two days' journey, but his eyes were resting on me, very expressively.

'Lili, my dear Lili, look up at me, you've kept me waiting too long!' His voice was quavering, and I wept on his chest. I cried my heart out, like a little girl, and he took my head in his trembling hands and kissed me as if to wipe my tears away. Our lips met, and we had a long, long kiss... we forgot everything around, we forgot the whole world, we only knew there were the two of us on this earth.

His first visit was very short. Nowhere in the hospital could he take a rest because it had no rooms for visitors, and the hotel he was staying at was very far away. Subsequently we met several times, and each time there was a happy reunion but a sad leavetaking. One day he said with a sob in his voice, 'Lili, let us be married, I cannot endure this situation any more...' and he burst into tears.

Really! It had occurred to me too that we ought to be married. I had been yearning for a man's caress, for a life with love, and above all, I wished I could be day and night with the one I cherished. But this dream would perhaps never come true, for so many obstacles still lay in the way. They were like insuperable peaks standing between us. Love did exist between us, and yet it was out of our reach. Such a love-without-love marathon was a perpetual torment.

I could only gaze at his picture, in the quietness of the night, with my tears to keep my company during my sleepless nights.

Beijing, People's Republic of China
November 1988

PREGNANCY AND SPINAL CORD INJURY*
Elizabeth Winkelaar

In July 1979, I was involved in a motor vehicle accident that left me paraplegic at T–8. Anyone who has experienced a spinal cord injury will agree that one of the outstanding concerns is how the subsequent handicap will affect his or her sexuality and ability to bear and raise children. I was married a year after my accident and in February 1982 gave birth to a baby boy, Christopher. Twenty-two months later I gave birth to a baby girl, Lesley. My experience in bearing and raising children has not been especially profound, but sharing my experiences with others might ease some doubts or answer some questions.

I have always lived in a small town, and our family doctor monitored my pregnancy and delivered our babies in our small-town hospital. My doctor would have preferred to do a Caesarian section, but I was anxious to deliver naturally and he agreed... Our first child weighted 7 lbs 3 oz... Our second weighed 5 lbs 13 oz and was delivered four weeks prematurely, with no forceps or episiotomy.

During my pregnancies I had no trouble with pressure sores, excess weight gain, blood pressure, bowel problems, or fluid retention. I did experience more incontinence than usual, especially during the first three months and the last few weeks. However, I stuck to my routine of intermittent catheterization.

With my second delivery, I was admitted to the hospital four weeks before my due date with a fairly severe bladder infection and fever, and two days after I was admitted I went into labour. My doctor felt that this infection, along with the fever, brought on the premature delivery.

One of my concerns before delivery was whether I would feel my contractions. I

have no motor control below my les but I do have some sensation and I could feel my contractions. I certainly knew when I was in labour, and I would describe the contractions as intense, although not painful. This made the deliveries enjoyable and I was very aware of the birth process. The labour of my first delivery lasted five hours, of my second two and a half hours.

Every pregnancy is different, just as every spinal cord injury is different, and I would advise anyone who wants to have a child to see a specialist and be monitored closely throughout the pregnancy. I feel that I was more lucky than smart. I was the first paraplegic to have a baby in our hospital and the first such delivery for my doctor. I had a different doctor for each delivery and both were conscientious...

The important thing is to get as much information as you can, don't be afraid to ask questions, and question the answers. If some aspect of delivery or post-natal care is important to you try every avenue to arrange things the way you want them.

MEDICATIONS AND PREGNANCY

Most women with spinal cord injuries must take some medication. It is the decision of the individual and the attending physician whether these medications should be continued during pregnancy.

The possible effects of a drug on the developing foetus must be considered and compared to the possible detriments to the mother if she discontinues a certain medication...

After Lesley was born, I found that I had begun to get contractures in my hamstrings, Achilles tendons, and at the level of my pelvis. It was impossible for me to straighten out my legs or lie flat on my stomach.

* Reprinted from *Rehabilitation Gazette*, Vol. 27, No. 2, 1986.

When Lesley was a year old, I was readmitted to my original rehabilitation centre (Lyndhurst, in Toronto) with these problems. I spent four months there, and through drug therapy and intensive physiotherapy we were able to reverse the contractures so I now have a fairly good range of motion. During that time, I began to use leg braces for the first time, which, at my level, I do not find practical for walking but extremely useful in controlling spasms, stretching out the legs, and feeling healthier in general...

I nursed Christopher for three months and Lesley for nine months quite successfully. I felt that it was less work, I enjoyed the closeness with the baby, and I had no complications to prevent me from nursing. I often lay down to nurse because I found it hard on my back to hold the baby in one position for that length of time. When I did nurse sitting up, I used a pillow to rest the baby on. With nursing, medications are again a consideration and this must be discussed with one's physician.

CHILDREN ADAPT EARLY

There are no simple answers on how to handle a baby, how to put it in a crib and take it out, and what is the best position for feeding. The balance and abilities of every mother are different, and every child develops at a different rate. As long as one considers safety at all times, every mother adapts to a situation; surprisingly early in their lives, every child also adapts. I found it interesting that, in comparison with other people's children, our babies developed good balance in the sitting position very early. This is one of many examples of how children adapt naturally to a parent's disability.

The only piece of special equipment that I needed or used was a change table made by my husband Felix. It is a good height for me, lower than the average change table, and I can wheel underneath it. There are shelves down the sides and a padded top...

Because our children are still so young, we do not know if my disability will affect them later in their childhood and adolescence. There is always a possibility that the attitude of their peers might cause them to regard their mother as 'different' in a negative way. I believe that a healthy attitude begets a healthy attitude, and if I can show my children that my physical limitations or differences do not prevent me from being a productive, loving, giving person, I think they will pass on this belief to their peers.

During the seven years I have been paraplegic, I have found that most life experiences take a little extra effort to be fulfilling and successful. Being a parent is a demanding but worthwhile role, and a spinal cord injury is certainly not a drawback to successful parenting. ●

A RESERVOIR OF STRENGTH*

Mary Hughes

During the summer of 1986, I had fusions performed at two levels in my cervical spine because of pinched nerves. When I woke up in the intensive care unit, I found I could not move my hands. Polio had left me with one leg paralysed and, now, thirty-five years later, the other leg seemed to be going downhill rather fast, but my arms had always been my salvation. Losing the use of my upper extremities had been my biggest fear. With the assistance of therapy, motion and strength returned to my hands, but I was discharged from the hospital with a sensory deficit in both hands. Sensory deficit also meant hand and arm strength were diminished when it came to performing chores involved in daily living.

* Reprinted from *Rehabilitation Gazette*, Vol. 27, No. 2, 1986.

I never expected to have both arms and hands, both legs, and my neck out of commission at the same time. I live alone and found caring for myself almost impossible. Tests showed there was no permanent damage to any nerves, but this didn't help me take a shower or prepare meals, even though it was comforting to hear. I turned to a home health care agency for assistance, but ran into a Nurse Ratchet type who referred to my brace as a 'limb' and tried to treat me as though my primary condition were mental retardation. Needless to say, our relationship was short-lived. Family and friends were of tremendous help, but my spirit sagged as I attempted to cope.

I had always managed before and was sure I could again, but the unexpected happened again; the hip that had been the donar site for bone for the fusion became extremely painful. I found I could not move without excruciating pain. I went from bad to worse in a few hours.

That night I found myself lying in bed crying because I felt I possessed no more coping ability, and because I was afraid. Was this a sample of what the future held for me. I was ready to give up and let others take charge of my life, something I had never before considered.

POSITIVE EXPERIENCE

I didn't give up and I don't know why. A horrible nightmare turned out to be a positive experience. I realize now that I was perhaps my own worst enemy, because I allowed myself to become so burdened with coping that I didn't think about available resources. I tried to shoulder everything and ended up almost losing everything – a waste of precious energy.

Being in control of one's life is a big issue for everyone, but I think it takes on greater significance for people who face the rigours of life in today's world with a physical disability. If we allow events to move us, if we find ourselves reacting to situations, I believe we are on a disastrous course. Granted, we cannot control all things, no one can, but to give up control in areas where it is possible to remain in charge is to open the door to depression and a feeling of greater helplessness, both of which only lead to greater problems.

I don't know what allowed me to tap into that reservoir of strength or where it came from, but I do know I have gained a greater feeling of confidence and control over my life that is invaluable. I work harder on applying the saying, 'It is not facts or events that upset man but the view he takes of them.' ●

1 'Women and disabilities: a national forum', *Entourage*, Vol. 3, No. 4, autumn 1988.
2 Ann Dornbrough, 'The secret handicap', UNESCO Features No. 763.
3 Sharon Mistler *International Rehabilitation Review* February 1977.
4 Balaknishna Venkatesh, 'Women with disabilities', appendix to *Beacon*, newsletter of Divine Light Trust for the Blind, October 1988.
5 Excerpt from an article by Debby Kaplan in *International Rehabilitation Review*, February 1977.
6 Excerpt from statement by the International Federation of Disabled Workers and Civilian Handicapped, Bonn, Germany.

5 CARE-GIVERS: IN THE SHADOW OF DISABILITY

Countless numbers of non-disabled people are also victims of disability – their lives deeply altered by the disability of others. . . these are the care-givers, and they are almost always women. For them, care-giving usually means lost opportunities for education and for employment outside the home. Taking care of a disabled family member leaves little time for social and leisure activities and dims the lives of these sometimes reluctant, sometimes resentful but usually resigned care-givers. . . they, too, need help.

DISABILITY CASTS ITS LONG SHADOW over the lives of non-disabled women – the care-givers – who are rarely given any alternative to accepting the restraining yoke that care-giving implies. They are forced to subordinate their own lives to this role, to give up opportunities for edu-cation and outside employment, to see social activities sharply curtailed by severe limitations of leisure time, to neglect the needs of non-disabled family members and to have the household budget strained by the disabled person's special needs.

A Japanese woman writes:

Several years ago, I was surprised when a physically handicapped male candidate for the Diet said at his supporters' meeting, 'I am looking for a woman for my wife who will take care of my toilette after my old mother passes away, because I have always been attended by my mother but she is getting old.' He never questioned the idea that a mother should devote her whole life to her son's care.[1]

Nor, apparently, did he question that a wife would not naturally take over the care-giving chores.

In a family with a disabled child or other family member, the special functions necessary for the care, education and social adjustment of disabled persons usually, in the absence of adequate services, are performed by the women or woman in the household, thus limiting in an unequal manner the rights and opportunities of the women concerned.[2]

Care-givers have needs of their own which have been too long ignored.

There are very few saints among the women who act as care-givers and, although for many care-giving is a labour of love, they are in some degree reluctant, resentful or merely resigned to this responsibility.

The World Conference to review the achievements of the United Nations Decade of Women called for measures which 'aim to protect those women who have a disabled person in their family, since such a burden weighs notably more heavily on women; such measures would enable them to lead as normal a life as possible.'[3]

CARE-GIVING SEEN AS 'DUTY' ☐ A recent survey undertaken by the ILO, on women with disabilities in six Asian countries,[4] included among its interviewees care-givers in each country. Findings of this survey showed, not surprisingly, that most care-givers were female family members who felt that the care of the disabled person was their 'duty'. Many felt inadequate to the task, that they needed at least basic training to carry out their care-giving chores efficiently, and that they also needed community support and financial help.

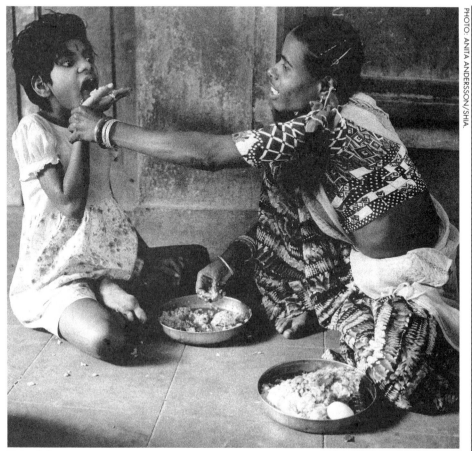

PHOTO: ANITA ANDERSSON/SHIA.

Madras Indian.

The report in the survey on Japan pointed out that even women with disabilities have, in come cases, assumed the duties of care-givers.

Today, the life expectancy of the Japanese is longer and Japan is a typical ageing society. The elderly and disabled people include severely disabled women and there is much need for home care and attendant services in ordinary family life. In that service market some women with disabilities have made attendant services their occupation.

To promote the establishment of non-governmental service agencies so that some disabled women are able to be careworkers efficiently, the Tokyo Metropolitan Government provided a fund of 20 million Yen (approximately US$140,200) to the Tokyo Community Welfare Promotion Foundation, and let the Foundation use the interest of the fund to support such non-governmental care agencies.[5]

In the Third World, women rarely have any option but to care for a disabled family member. Many care-giver respondents in developing countries within the ILO survey freely admitted that they found their disabled charges difficult and that, if the opportunity were offered, they would not oppose their being transferred to institutional care.

An intriguing new dimension to care-giving has recently appeared in the USA. A programme is being carried out at the Helping Hands Training Center in Brighton, Massachusetts, to train monkeys to assist quadriplegics with a few of their daily needs! And apparently the monkeys are doing very well indeed.

FOOD FOR THOUGHT *
Janet Finch

In the last five years, carers have become visible. It is sometimes difficult to remember that even the word 'carers' has only passed into our language very recently, when researchers and others began to uncover just how much unpaid work is being done by people who care for dependent members of their own family. Politicians and government departments also started to wake up to the value of this work in their planning of health and welfare services.

It is now recognized, in policy debate and in service planning, that carers too have needs; hence, respite care, support groups, the careful planning of care packages, and so on. One of the few policy issues upon which all major political parties agree is that these developments are the right way forward for the future: we need more community care and it needs to make serious attempts to 'support the carers'.

Is this a major and positive step foward? Of course, in some ways it certainly is. For anyone who has spent the last twenty years taking daily responsibility for the health and welfare of an elderly mother or a mentally handicapped son, there have certainly been improvements: some practical support, possibly a little extra money

in the form of invalid care allowance, and, perhaps most of all, the recognition that you are doing a very important job, making an important contribution to the way that society cares for its members.

But looked at from a different angle, the picture is not so positive. The cosy agreement that community care is the way forward has been challenged in the past only by the voices of feminists, who have asked whether continuing to rely on unpaid care is not, in effect, a way to ensure that women remain unequal in our society. That question is still very relevant.

SEPARATE WELFARE STATE

The introduction in recent years of more services that support family carers – both practically and financially – has been a marginal contribution by comparison with the value of the work that they perform. By counting the number of hours that carers of elderly people spend in looking after them, and then costing this out at the price of a home help's wage, researchers at the Family Policy Studies Centre have estimated that the cost is equal to that for the total for the statutory health and social services for over-75-year-olds.

Carers are, in other words, providing a separate welfare state on the same scale as that for which we pay our taxes. The great majority of the people who provide this care are women. There seems general agreement that at least three-quarters of unpaid family carers are women, and that men normally become carers only of their wives, whereas women take this role on for other members of their family, as well as for their husbands.

The support that carers receive pales into insignificance compared to the massive range of services that women carers provide.

---

* Reprinted from *Carelink*, No. 2, summer 1987. Janet Finch is senior lecturer in social administration at the University of Lancaster, U.K.

The most common response to this is that it is perfectly all right: there is no problem about women providing this large quantity of unpaid care, because they actually want to do it. Of course, no one would wish to prevent someone caring for a relative if they want to; but the problem is, how do we know if they want to do it? And what does 'want to' actually mean?

The idea that someone does anything because they want to implies that they have some choice: that there are other realistic alternatives, but the carer has rejected them and chosen to do the work herself. For most people that simply does not reflect the reality of how they become unpaid carers.

Unless they are in the position to pay for private care – either in the home or residential care – the chances are that no other options are available, or at least none that the carer, and their relative, can accept as a comfortable and dignified way to live.

Unfortunately, the stream of recent policy documents promoting community care continues to assume that not only do individuals become carers because they want to, but also that wanting to provide unpaid care for your relatives is a natural part of family life. This point is frequently regarded as so obvious that it does not even need to be stated. But is it obvious?

'I DON'T WANT TO BE A BURDEN'

We know that people's feelings about their relatives are very personal and have a long history, stretching back into childhood, often containing many negative as well as positive elements. Clearly, an unquestioning desire to provide care for your relatives is not a universal emotion. But even where relationships are warm and positive, should we assume that people automatically regard it as a necessary part of that relationship that they should provide nursing and domestic services on a daily basis,

possibly for many years?

That assumption flies in the face of most of the research published since the 1950s. On the family relationships of older people, for example, the strong message is that old people like to have warm relationships with their relatives, but ideally they do not want to live together and they do not want to impose upon them too much. The phrase, 'I don't want to be a burden', is so familiar to anyone who works in this field... but it is a serious statement about what family relationships ought to be like. It reflects, quite accurately, research evidence about what people today feel to be the proper and desirable way of conducting family relationships. There is no real basis for assuming that unpaid care – especially if it becomes very demanding – is generally seen as a natural and unquestioned part of family life.

So why do such large numbers of women continue caring for their relatives? Why don't they give up and refuse to do it any longer? Some people may indeed worry that this is about to happen, which would then leave all those health and welfare plans, which depend on the expansion of community care, looking rather thin,

But I do not believe that this is about to happen. First, despite the expansion of work for women over recent years – mostly part-time, of course – our society is still basically organized on the principle that most people live in families in which there is a male breadwinner, and that women are financially dependent. Women still do not have working lives as wage earners in the same way that men do, and to that extent they are 'available' to care in a way which men are not, and I see little sign of any radical change in the foreseeable future.

Second, women's social identities and personal qualities are still very different from men's; women are perceived as 'people who care' in a way that men do not

67

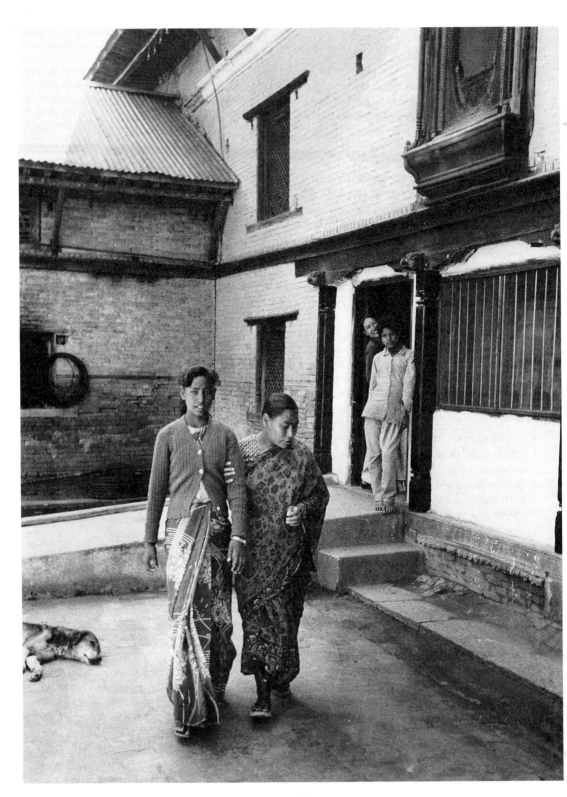

need to be. To be someone whom others see as 'uncaring' damages the social status of a woman much more seriously than that of a man, and women usually have fewer alternative sources of status and self-esteem. It therefore becomes extremely difficult for women not to provide care for a relative when everyone around is saying that community care is a good idea and that it is most natural for dependent people to be with their families.

Third, the lack of choice of alternative forms of care that would be acceptable to all parties means that potential carers are forced to make a stark choice: either provide it yourself, or your relative will end up with a form of care that is inadequate, or that they find unacceptable, perhaps even shameful. That puts powerful pressure on to women particularly, especially if the relationship with the person in need of care is warm and close. Faced with the inadequate alternatives available, they will 'naturally' feel that they 'want to' care, but that does not mean that they think this is fundamentally the most desirable solution. For all these reasons, I believe that women will continue to be carers, but at the same time their position in society as men's dependants and the supporters and servicers of other people is thereby being reinforced.

Ironically even those very services that have begun to support carers actually also maintain women's position in the division of caring labour, because they provide just enough respite from the work women do to ensure that they do not give up or crack up.

Of course these policies do provide personal support, and I certainly would not wish to return to the days when carers were invisible and entirely unsupported. Nevertheless, if we recognize that they also reinforce gender inequalities, we have to face some difficult moral and political choices. ●

WOMEN ASSISTING DISABLED PERSONS *
Dra Teresa Selli Serra

When we say that 10 per cent of the world population is disabled – which means about 500 million disabled persons – we often forget that there are at least 500 million women in the world who in one way or another are involved in the care of their disabled family members.

Society, in fact, has always taken for granted that the care of infants, sick, elderly and disabled persons is a family responsibility, but in practice such responsibility, especially in the modern urban nuclear family, falls mostly on women.

What I want to stress here is the importance of offering a real, free choice to both the disabled person and the woman of the family who is expected to assist him or her.

In fact, the type of relationship that exists between disabled persons and their carers or helpers is a very delicate one. If the woman assisting a disabled person does not freely choose to do it, or if the disabled person does not freely accept her service, the relationship between the two (obliged to live together) can have a very negative influence on both of them.

It is therefore essential for the general well-being and mental health of both parties that a real choice is at the base of their partnership. But in order to choose freely, a variety of options must be available and society should be responsible for offering different types of solutions to suit individual needs.

Until now, the only option offered in many countries has been the service given by women in the family. In some countries legislation even obliges families to

* Reprinted from Proceedings of the 16th World Congress of Rehabilitation International, Tokyo, 1988. Dra Serra is President of the Italian Spastic Society and National Secretary of Rehabilitation International, Italy.

care for their dependent members. In some others legislation gives incentives or pays housewives for the assistance they provide – but this is not a satisfactory approach to the problem; a variety of solutions is necessary.

Unfortunately society rarely offers different options. Even where new approaches and alternative solutions have been offered, there is always the danger in many countries that recurrent economic crises may result in the task of caring for disabled persons again becoming a family responsibility.

In the past few years, I have followed with great interest the growth of the Independent Living Movement. Their views – from the perspective of disabled persons – are that such persons want to make their own choices about their lives and to be responsible for their own personal assistance service. They consider that personal assistance is the key to independent living and they define independent living as the ability to exercise choices. They want to choose whom they want as assistants and in my opinion they are right.

From the perspective of women, the problem is exactly the same. Women should not be or should not feel morally obliged to assist a disabled relative. They should be given a choice and, if they want to act in this capacity, they must be certain that they may count on family supportive services when they need help. Otherwise, in the long run even the best relationship may disintegrate and both members suffer acutely.

SHUNNING THE TRADITIONAL ROLE

I belong to that generation of mothers of spastic children who, during the 1950s, started to refuse the traditional role of care-givers but at the same time refused to put their handicapped children in an institution and forget about them. This course

was often suggested at that time by doctors, who later admittedly recognized that 'if parents had not pushed them [the doctors] into doing something, they would probably have continued to consider cerebral palsied children as incurable'.

These words were said to me in 1953 in England, where I took my cerebral palsied child for early treatment. A now famous British doctor pushed and encouraged me to do in my country what parents had done in England and in other countries. Following his advice, one year later I founded the Italian Spastics Association.

November 1954 seems to have been a fortunate period for the cerebral palsy movement: two other mothers, without knowing each other, started cerebral palsy organizations in European countries. Similar moves had already occurred in the USA and in other countries around the world. Some years later the Director of Special Education in Oslo said: 'We had mothers in different countries who would stop at nothing, trying again and again to convince physicians to study their children and eventually find ways of helping them.'

My experience in England was very useful and it helped me not to seclude within my family circle a problem that had to be shared with others, not only with those who had the same problem but also with those unaware of it. The tendency of families with handicapped children was to see their problem as an individual, and not a social, problem.

Disability was experienced as a dramatic event concerning only the parents and particularly the mother. It was something that could not even be mentioned to neighbours, either because parents were afraid of misunderstanding, pity and prejudices, or because they themselves had feelings of guilt or shame deriving from a certain type of education or cultural attitude that considered handicapped people to be inferior, as a burden on society or even as the fruit of sin.

PARENTS ORGANISE GROUPS

Families frequently resigned themselves to accept a physician's verdict that the condition was allegedly incurable and followed his or her advice to put the child in a nursing home. Those who refused to accept such advice ended up upsetting their entire lives in order to be able to care for their child at home because there were no alternative solutions. The fact that mothers and parents of the 1950s refused the old schemes and started first, to talk among themselves about their mutual problems and, later, to go openly out to inform public opinion about their needs and to ask for adequate rehabilitation services represented a turning point and made it possible to shift from the initial resigned and passive attitude of families, but particularly of mothers, to a more active and dynamic role.

Where public authorities did not take responsibility to provide them directly, parents groups themselves started to organize the new alternative services which, at that time, were considered the best. I refer to day centres as an alternative to nursing homes, and day or boarding schools (even special ones) as alternatives to the previously enforced illiteracy of so many handicapped children.

Exactly thirty years have elapsed since those first efforts. Now, many of the mothers of the 1950s have had the satisfaction of seeing their handicapped children grow up to become independent, self-sufficient adults. Other mothers, however (and I know quite a few of them), have seen their problems become more serious as time passes, either because their children, although chronologically adults, remain in need of constant assistance or because, although grown-up and capable of participating in social and economic activities, they are physically dependent on others for their daily needs and mobility.

These mothers are still fighting for family-supportive services and for alternative solutions to nursing homes or mental hospitals, where their adult, dependent children can live, especially if parents can no longer care for them. The need for such alternative solutions, for new ways of providing supported living conditions, is increasingly felt.

In various parts of the world there is a growing movement: the Independent Living Movement in which young disabled persons are very active. Mothers and their severely disabled adult offspring cannot be left alone in this struggle. Solidarity with these families is essential and it also represents a preventive measure – otherwise there is a risk, in the long run, that all family members may become physically, psychologically or economically destroyed, despite the best family attitude towards involvement with its disabled member.

It is in the interests of the community to avoid that risk by making more and more of these alternative solutions available from the beginning of adulthood, in order that both disabled persons and their families may have the freedom to choose the type of living conditions best suited to their individual needs. This type of solution would meet the need of young and adult disabled persons to choose freely, or to adjust gradually to, the living conditions that will best suit them instead of being compelled to prolong their adolescence indefinitely by spending all their lives with their parents.

But, above all, this type of solution would satisfy the need and the right of parents to spend the last years of their lives in serenity and to die in peace. Elderly parents, and especially elderly mothers (who often remain alone to cope with their grown-up dependent disabled children either because they are widows or separated from their husbands) have very often dedicated their entire lives to caring for their child who 'never grew up' and they have reached a stage at which not only are they no longer sufficiently physically fit to assist their children but also, and primarily, they are worried about their children's future. Their only wish is to know that there will be a suitable solution for the care of their children when they, themselves, are no longer alive.

1 Yayori Matsui, 'UN Decade of Women and Special Concern on Disabled Women', summary report.
2 Susan R. Hammerman, 'Women and disability', Rehabilitation International Conference on Women with Disabilities, New York, February 1986.
3 Ibid.
4 *Dispelling the Shadows of Neglect: a survey on women with disabilities in six Asian and Pacific countries*, ILO, Geneva, June 1989.
5 Dr Y. Kojima, 'Strategies to improve socio-vocational integration of disabled women in Japan'. Written from research sponsored by the ILO.

GROWING OLDER – A TIME TO ENDURE... OR ENJOY?

Failing eyesight, loss of hearing, frequent illness and, perhaps most debilitating of all, loneliness, can effectively tarnish the 'golden years' of old age. These problems of ageing that people without handicap face carry the further threat of disability. This is especially true for women who not only tend to live longer than men but, in the age of the nuclear family, usually cope with these problems alone.

As women who have lived with disability grow older, these infirmities common to ageing women may become all the more serious due to disability. As their limited capacities diminish with age, any degree of independence they may have achieved is in jeopardy.

A 'MYSTIQUE OF AGE' denies personhood to people older than sixty – ageism in society discriminates against the elderly just as sexism discriminates against women, according to Betty Friedan, whose book *The Feminine Mystique* gave so much impetus to the feminist movement in the United States.

Betty Friedan has recently taken up the cause of older women and the problems that beset them as they get older. Ten years ago she brushed aside requests that she use her considerable influence in the women's movement to arouse more concern for ageing women. 'I had the same view of ageing as everyone else in America,' she has said. 'You know, poor things, dreary. Not me.'[1] But she listened and her attitude changed. Her about-face inspired a new book, *The Fountain of Age*, which she hopes will do for the elderly what *The Feminine Mystique* did for women.

> Women are living longer than men and, as they age, become especially prone to disabling disorders.

Betty Friedan's enthusiastic involvement in their welfare is good news for elderly women in the USA – they need all the help they can get. Nearly three-fourths of the country's residents in nursing homes are women; of the 29 million Americans who are aged sixty-five or older, 21 million are women; of the nearly 9 million Americans aged sixty-five and older living alone, more than 80 per cent are women; the typical elderly person living alone is a widow, poor and in her eighties.

The phenomenon of an ageing population is not confined to the USA – the trend is apparent in most advanced industrialised countries – people are living longer and women are living longer than men. In the final analysis, old age and its pitfalls concern primarily women.

Coco Chanel, the high priestess of French fashion, has been quoted as saying that 'after forty-five, a woman can no longer call herself young'. Midlife is a watershed in a woman's existence – it is then that the spectre of ageing with its possibilities of chronic illness, disability and decline comes into sharper focus.

Women with disabilities at the midlife transition period face the possibility of three-fold discrimination based on sex, disability and age.

Pre-existence or sudden occurrence of disability during this period may have ramifications for the individual woman. For example, a woman disabled

73

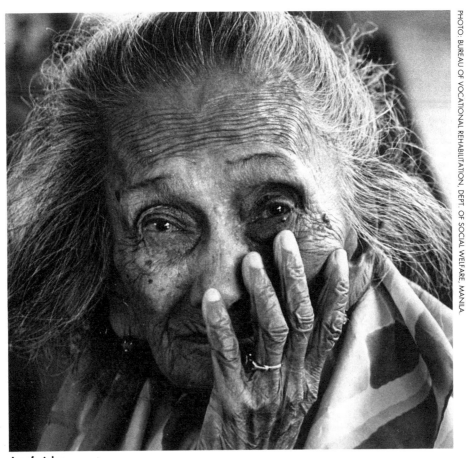

PHOTO: BUREAU OF VOCATIONAL REHABILITATION, DEPT. OF SOCIAL WELFARE, MANILA.

Age of wisdom.

early in life may have resolved the issues of body image, a unique means of completing tasks of daily living, personal coping with mechanisms, and social interaction... The recently-disabled woman's feelings about her new status will depend on her self image, support system, social and physical environment and the creative coping abilities that she can mobilise to adjust psychologically and physically.[2]

PROBLEMS OF AGEING □ As the years go by, ageing women become especially prone to disabling disorders such as arthritis, osteoporosis (fragile bones), incontinence, diabetes, cancer, depression and paraphrenia (mental disorders).

Furthermore, experts add:

The prolongation of life presents a new variety of health and welfare problems. Studies have shown that the ageing person is, in general, confronted with giving up social roles and relationships, increased social isolation, increased anxiety about income and over possible loss of health and possible incapacity. These changes may occur at a time when the older person's resources may be rapidly declining and dependency increasing... Since women have more chronic diseases, live longer than men, and have lower mortality rates for most of the causes of death, they need a more comprehensive range of health care services...

The need for long-term care (LTC) services is expected to grow dramatically in the near future in the United States. The most dramatic changes in population will be among those 85 years of age or older who will increase at the rate of 18 per cent or greater every five years between 1980 and 2000. The projected need for increased LTC services is projected not only on the increased number of very elderly but also on the number of elderly having disabilities. Elderly women dominate both groups...

Older women are far more likely than older men to live alone and often lack adequate support systems. This isolation makes the treatment of physical and mental illness more difficult.

It may also be a precipitating factor related to the increased number of women who are institutionalised. Older women in poor health find it more difficult to stay in the community since they have fewer social and financial resources than men. They also have more functional limitations, and more problems with daily living which contribute to institutionalisation.[3]

Studies have shown, however, that many elderly persons can manage successfully at home, if they are given appropriate services. Some communities in the USA are experimenting with home and community-based aid as alternatives to nursing-home care, using day-care centres, homemaker and home health services and self-care.

Day-care centres cater for frail, moderately handicapped or slightly confused older persons who need care during the day, whilst homemaker and home health services are carried out in the home by women skilled both as homemakers and care-givers.

CHALLENGING IMAGES OF 'HELPLESSNESS' ☐

The self-care programme, in addition to training elderly women to take more responsibility for their own health by preventing, detecting and treating common illness and injury, also aims at changing their image of being helpless and dependent, which is one of the manifestations of ageism and sexism. Such stereotyping is, unfortunately, too often present in the medical profession, which has shown negative attitudes towards the elderly.

A study of medical care of the aged in the United States has shown that such care is characterised by negativism, defeatism and professional antipathy... Sexist stereotypes influence the medical profession to believe that illness and discomfort observed in women are largely due to psychological origins. On the other hand, women with certain problems that have psychological causes, such as loneliness and poor self-image, which do not need medical treatment are often referred to health care services... Two studies of medical and doctoral students found that the students preferred not to work with older adults. A study of nursing students also found similar preferences.[4]

Efforts are being made by many health professions' schools to nip this negativism in the bud. For example, a Gerontology Internship Program sponsored by Cornell University Medical College in the USA involves students in the daily lives of their older patients. That such programmes are urgently needed is vividly demonstrated by the shocking situation uncovered in spring 1989 in a Vienna hospital where, apparently over a period of several years, older patients had been systematically murdered by hospital workers who said that the patients were 'too old or disagreeable'.

Indifference among health care workers is also found in the UK where:

Disabled, elderly women were too often left alone, with health and social services only getting involved when there was a crisis... and the services they then receive tend to be inappropriate or insensitively administered... Some health workers are accused of inflexibility and narrowness of attitude towards women in wheelchairs: being in a wheelchair becomes the condition. If you complain about other things that are wrong with you, they say, what do you expect?[5]

TOO OLD FOR MOBILITY BENEFIT □
In a survey undertaken by the Greater London Association for Disabled People (GLAD), the Mobility Allowance, a tax-free cash benefit of £21.40 a week, came under heavy fire from ageing disabled women.

While the allowance is intended to help severely disabled people become more mobile – it can be used in any way the recipient chooses, for example for buying or hiring a car, taxis, paying for a holiday, buying or running an electric wheelchair – in order to qualify for it you must be unable or virtually unable to walk and you must be *under 66 years of age*.

Considering that the most common form of disability is arthritis, which is also very common amongst ageing women, it can be seen that many women with worsening disabilities are excluded from claiming this potentially liberating benefit.... If a handicapped person over 66 years old wants an electric wheelchair and does not qualify for Mobility Allowance because of her age and cannot otherwise afford one, her only option may be to get one through a charity. However, she may not be able to do this or may not be inclined to do so. Finally, she may be left unaided.... Many women with disabilities have not been outside their home for years. The attendant psychological problems of extreme isolation frequently make even more difficult finding solutions for problems that are relatively easy to handle about physical disability.... Indeed, the underlying rationale behind the age limit seems to be that 'after all, you can expect disability in old age'.[6]

It must be recognised that the health needs of older women may differ according to the age group to which they belong, 65–74, 75–84 and over 85 years. The needs of very elderly women, whose risks are immediate and linked to longterm care issues, are different from those of women in the 65–74-year-old group who may be old in years, but who function at a high level until they come up against health and/or economic problems. Other variables that may affect an older woman's health include her educational status, ethnic or cultural origins, socioeconomic status and geographic location.

There is, of course, another group of ageing women for whom growing older is a double source of worry – the women care-givers. Mothers who have always looked after a severely handicapped child not only dread their own possible incapacity in future due to ageing, but are also haunted by the worry, 'What will happen when I die?'

Women should be able to enjoy old age, not merely endure it. It can be a time of sharing and of freedom from personal insecurities, and, for some, a time when new activities or experiences may be tried out.

To help make old age truly 'the golden years' for women, health professions' schools would need to give more attention to the older years of life and expand their curricula, taking into account the following issues:

● There is a need to integrate geriatric and gerontological (ageing) issues, particularly those of older women, into every health profession's school curriculum.
● Intensive, short-term, continuing education courses are needed to update the knowledge and skills of the current faculty, particularly in the area of geriatric assessment.

- Schools should stress the need for interdisciplinary collaboration in dealing with issues of ageing, by providing resources for the purpose.
- Recruitment efforts should be intensified among minority groups in the health professions since the number of minority elderly women is likely to increase dramatically during the next decade and since minority groups are under-represented in this area.
- There is a need to give support to clinical training programmes in mental health and ageing, and to develop training sites for clinical experience with elderly women, particularly in the community, as well as in hospitals and nursing homes.[7]

At the same time, rather than see older women continue to stand idly by, passively awaiting inevitable decline, health professionals should help and encourage them to become actively engaged in their own health care, and especially to:

- be able to distinguish the physical and mental changes accompanying the normal ageing process from those that would be considered abnormal. This would include dispelling certain popular myths about ageing;
- seek timely help from an appropriate health professional, including preventive care;
- communicate effectively with health professionals – asking the right questions, understanding health information;
- focus on the importance of maintaining a healthy lifestyle in disease prevention.[8]

In declaring war against ageism, Betty Friedan drew on the work of the poet Dylan Thomas when she said, 'We will not go gently into the good night or sit in rocking chairs in these nursing homes.' Thomas's original poem reads, in part:

**Do not go gentle into that good night,
Old age should burn and rave at close of day;
Rage, rage against the dying of the light.**

Surely this can be more inspiring than to hear 'After all, one can only expect disability in old age.'

LIVING INDEPENDENTLY AT EIGHTY-FIVE*
Dorothea Richtberg

Each summer, my family would leave the hot city of Manhattan for a glorious retreat at a farm boarding-house in upper New York State, where, in 1907, I contracted polio at the age of five. Operations, braces, and crutches helped me to walk so that I could attend high school and college, including postgraduate work in microbiology.

I have a most supportive family and was lucky to have the opportunity to travel to Europe and Alaska, where I felt like a pioneer.

In 1930, I had difficulty walking and underwent two operations that helped me achieve greater stability and allowed me to discard the supportive shoes, although I still needed a crutch and a cane.

I was working as a microbiologist at Mt Sinai Hospital in 1931, when a physical therapist showed me Sister Kenny's method of exercise. The exercises greatly improved my walking and I still do some of them today.

I retired in 1963, and moved to Princeton, New Jersey, with my sister. In Princeton, I learned Braille and worked for the Princeton Recording for the Blind.

---

* Reprinted from *Rehabilitation Gazette*, Vol. 27, No. 2, 1986.

Thirteen years later, we moved to Medford Leas, a retirement community with about five hundred residents and a medical centre for eighty residents. I am involved in several of the 70 or so committees organised by the residents. At Medford Leas I had post-polio complications resulting in complete paralysis of my 'good' left leg. Two years ago, I pulled muscles in my good left shoulder, necessitating complete reliance on a wheelchair. Nevertheless, I am happy that at eighty-five I am still independent enough to care for myself, to stay active, and to do all the things I enjoy doing. ●

1 Molly Sinclair, 'Betty Friedan takes on "age mystique", *International Herald Tribune*, 25–26 February 1989.
2 Kay Harris Kriegsman and Sue Gregman, 'Women with disabilities at midlife', *Rehabilitation Counselling Bulletin*, December 1965.
3 *Women's Health – Report of the Public Health Task Force on Women's Health Issues*, US Department of Health and Human Services, Washington, D.C.
4 Ibid.
5 Susan Holland, 'Women, disability and ageing', *GLAD Quarterly*, winter 1986 (published by Greater London Association for Disabled).
6 Ibid.
7 *Women's health – Report of the Public Health Task Force on Women's Health Issues*, US Department of Health and Human Services.
8 Ibid.

NEW HORIZONS: TAKING CONTROL

After failing to get jobs at local factories and offices because of her disability, a woman who was born with fingers and toes missing has built a thriving garment-making business in a small Philippine village where unemployment is endemic... A sailing vessel that crossed the Atlantic Ocean in 1988 had a seven-member crew, four of whom were disabled, and one of the disabled crew members was a woman.

SUCH ACHIEVEMENTS BY DISABLED WOMEN show a determination to leave the claustrophobic world of disability – a determination that must be fostered and encouraged, among all women with disabilities, by helping them to find their place in the non-disabled world.

AN INNOVATIVE PHILIPPINE PROGRAMME CREATES ENTREPRENEURS*

━━━━━━━━━━━━━ David Kinley

The Philippine fishing town of Morong (population 29,000) provides no exception to the chronic unemployment that plagues many small communities surrounding Manila. Yet Amelita de la Vega's streetside garment shop is crowded with employees, its Singer sewing machines whirring busily almost every steamy evening.

By any yardstick, Mrs de la Vega is a extraordinarily successful entrepreneur. Her homespun manufacturing business, appraised at $160,000, employs at least thirty men and women. She travels weekly to Manila to deal with major exporters, and even sub-contracts additional production from other new shops that she has helped establish around Morong. Her baby clothes and women's shirts and blouses are eagerly sought by buyers from New York, Panama and Hawaii.

Mrs de la Vega's rise from poverty to business mogul is a source of hope for a Philippine economy long wracked by recession, trade deficits and widespread unemployment. What makes her story more extraordinary is that she belongs to a most disadvantaged and forgotten class of the Philippine poor, the physically disabled. Since birth, Mrs de la Vega has faced daily survival with fingers and toes missing from both her hands and feet.

While exceptional, the experience of Amelita de la Vega is not unique. She is one of almost 1,500 disabled people throughout the Philippines who have been helped by an innovative rehabilitation project supported by the United Nations Development Programme (UNDP) and executed by the ILO, together with the Philippine government.

Mrs de la Vega's successul venture into the international garment business had its origins in that project. Just four years ago, she worked in her home while raising two children on the small income of her husband, a tricycle taxidriver. Though she'd acquired some business skills in college, she was routinely turned away from jobs at local factories and offices because of her disability.

'I was bored at home and wanted to help my husband and kids,' says Mrs de la Vega. 'One day a project volunteer came to my home and encouraged me to talk with a neighbour, who offered to lend me her old sewing machine'.

---

* Reprinted, in a condensed version, from *World Development*, United Nations Development Progamme, September 1988.

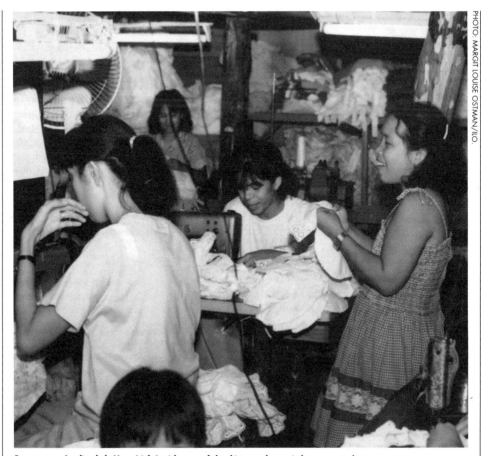

PHOTO: MARGIT LOUISE OSTMAN/ILO.

Entrepreneur Amelita de la Vega (right) with some of the thirty employees in her garment shop.

RAPID EXPANSION

The first night, Mrs de la Vega carefully dissected one of her small son's shirts. Manipulating scissors and paper with the palms of her hands and her thumbs, she created a paper pattern. Buying material in the marketplace, she began using the old sewing machine to fashion several shirts daily, no easy task for a person lacking fingers. Her colourful new shirts quickly became recognised in the Morong market for their high quality and competitive price.

Mrs de la Vega poured her earnings back into her business and soon began to build an inventory of stock and materials,

hiring and training other seamstresses – including other disabled people – and buying more used sewing machines. Through the help of her neighbour, she built contacts with exporters in Manila. Her business, helped by energetic management, grew rapidly into today's success story.

In contrast to conventional approaches to aiding the disabled through special centres, this experimental project places particular emphasis on volunteerism, community involvement, and economic self-reliance.

Amelita de la Vega provides testimony to the project's basic working principles: that disabled people are capable of useful, income-earning work if given a chance. ●

THE ONLY FEMALE ON BOARD *

Elisabeth Ryden

The only girl in the crew on a schooner crossing the Atlantic Ocean? Not even in my wildest imagination would I have thought it would happen to me, but it did.

The crew of seven persons was mixed, but most of us were physically handi-capped. I, a thalidomide-injured young woman with short arms, now had the chance to show what I could do. I had to manage.

The departure from Newport was delayed by bad weather. We were inter-viewed by the press and TV, and felt both embarrassed and pleased to be able to talk about the purpose of this voyage and the situation for handicapped people in general.

After ten days of waiting, we could finally depart. Escorted by a ship filled with new-won friends and a TV team we left Newport. It was glorious!

NO SPECIAL TREATMENT

But that night it wasn't glorious at all. Swells made almost the whole crew feel sick, and I spent hours by the gunwale. Maybe that was good because I never got sick again during the whole journey. Sometimes I felt that the whole crew had decided to give me extra tough jobs just to show that girls are not to be specially treated.

Normally there is a warm, south-east wind on the Atlantic Ocean from May through July. Not this year. We were sub-jected to several severe storms with cold, north-west winds. The winds were so strong that we were thrown out of the Gulf Stream, which we were to have fol-lowed during much of the voyage. Waves as big as three-storey houses piled up around us and we felt really small.

The ship was not completely well-adjusted to all types of handicaps, and

after a week it seemed like I had played a marathon match in rugby without protec-tion. Bruises everywhere! It took me a while to find out how to get a firm grip and not be thrown around while the ship was tossing. When I was just a little girl, my mother had started to improve my sense of balance – I was rather good at skipping as a child – and I have kept myself fit through exercise. This was a tremendous help to me now, as I couldn't use my arms as counter-balances.

Everything was on a schedule except the washing of clothes, which was done with rain or sea water. We spent our days cooking, sleeping or being at the helm, and we often lost any conception of time. We washed ourselves when the sun was shining – not too often. Otherwise it was cold. When I was at the helm at night, I wore eight sweaters and a jacket and I still froze!

After three weeks we came to the Azores. I was excited to disembark. How were we going to be met? We engendered both distrust and astonishment.

We had apparently entered an area that had previously been reserved for he-men, luxury yachts and adventurers. But when we told them about our hardships and lis-tened to their stories, we were able to meet as equals and have a beer together.

Great demands are made in living so close together and being so dependent on one another for such a long time. Sometimes it would have been nice to have been treated like a fragile flower, but that was obviously out of the question. Every hand was needed. At home I had seen myself on deck in the sun, sometimes taking small dips in the ocean. The reality was different: the second day I saw a 10 metre long shark just outside the ship. I immediately decided to give up the idea of dips. Later, seeing a man-of-war with 10-

* Reprinted from *Vox Nostra* (Disabled People's International), No. 1, 1989.

metre long tentacles that can easily kill a person made me absolutely sure there was no time for dips.

We felt we had achieved a great deal and shown that people with handicaps can participate in physically demanding activities. It was an unforgettable trip with many fantastic experiences. As it was the first time a journey like this has been made, we felt great to have managed it, especially with the terrible weather. I hope this means a new start for handicapped people. ●

THE IMPORTANCE OF SELF-HELP □

The recent accomplishments of these two disabled women, Elisabeth and Amelita, are as strikingly different as their origins – one helping to crew a sailing vessel on a pleasure trip across the Atlantic Ocean, and the other starting a business from scratch in a steamy fishing town in the Philippines. Although their lives are far apart, this wide gulf emphasizes the importance of self-help in a disabled woman's life and what can be accomplished by initiative and determination.

In recent years, there has been a noticeable groundswell in the self-help movement among women with disabilities, but as is usually the case, progress toward independent living is confined almost exclusively to the developed countries.

Personal achievement – based on self-confidence – can open up new horizons for motivated women with disabilities.

Experience has proven beyond doubt that the force of self-help is vitally important in enhancing the process of achieving full participation and equality in society for the disabled community. From this premise it follows that women with disability should be fully and equally involved in this self-help process in order to achieve full participation and equality in society along with their male counterparts.

The irony of the situation is that in the case of a woman with disability, the basic human rights of education, training, economic independence, participation in society, mobility and access to places are much more violated as compared to a man with disability – and yet she remains deprived of adequate involvement and representation in the self-help movement, which is the best and quickest way to redress her problems. This is due partly to socio-cultural, attitudinal and structural barriers and partly to male domination and prejudice against her right to equality in this field, so that no incentive or encouragement is given her to help her overcome the obstacles in her way.

Of course the situation of disabled women differs not only in the developed and developing worlds but also from region to region due to social, economic, religious and political factors. In the developed world the disabled woman has the facility of disability allowance to permit some degree of economic self-sufficiency; of education which is compulsory; of training; and, as a result of education and training, better preparation for a wider range of employment.

She has access to special equipment designed to help her function as normally as possible despite her disability. Environmental adjustments give her access to places of work, education, entertainment and public utilities. Today, disabled people are also gradually achieving access to independent living.

However, as far as the developing world is concerned, there is rarely, if ever, any disability allowance, or environmental adjustment. Very few women have access to education or training and a very limited number are employed – generally in poorly paid jobs. In view of the situation of women in

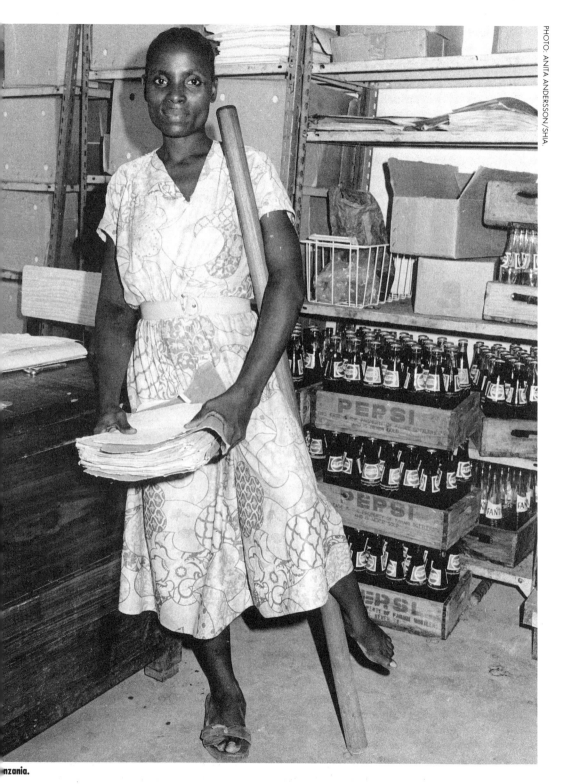

nzania.

83

general, and of women with disability in particular, it is not difficult to understand why they do not have an opportunity of involving themselves in self-help movements, particularly on the local and national levels.[1]

LEADERSHIP TRAINING SEMINARS ☐
Constructive efforts are being made, however, to open up new horizons for women with disability in developing countries, aimed at involving them in their own destiny. To this end, Disabled People's International (DPI) Asia–Pacific Region organized the first of a series of leadership training seminars for disabled women in Seoul, Republic of Korea, in October 1986. It was followed by a seminar in Mauritius in September 1987 under the auspices of DPI African Council and the Standing Committee on the Affairs of Women with Disability (SCAWD), and attended by women with disabilities from all parts of Africa. In December 1987 a leadership training seminar for South Asian women, held in Islamabad, Pakistan, which DPI Asia–Pacific also sponsored, included for the first time representatives from the usually neglected categories of disability – those suffering from mental, speech and hearing handicaps.

Included among the wide range of topics covered in these seminars is the organization and management of self-help movements. The leadership training received by the disabled women participants is intended to ensure the formation of grass-roots self-help movements by the participants when they return home.

Strategies that will enhance the development of leadership in women with disability may be listed as follows:

Leadership training seminars at the macro-level should pass on to the grassroots to benefit larger numbers of women with disability at the local level. Unless leadership is effective at the community level real change in the status of women with disability

cannot be achieved.

Information literature should be widely distributed but access to it is worthwhile only if translations in the various national languages are available. It is recommended that DPI Headquarters/ regional offices, in collaboration with UN agencies, may serve as clearing-houses for printed and audio-visual material.

Supportive media communication at national level to increase the public awareness of all aspects of disability is absolutely essential. Women with disability – in fact, all disabled persons – should not be depicted as passive recipients of benefits but as playing contributing and active roles.

Self-help organisations of disabled persons should launch frequent membership campaigns to motivate more and more women with disability to become members. Membership should be open to all, without educational or social status discrimination. When this type of membership is available, uneducated and low-income group disabled women will be encouraged to join existing organisations.

The formation of Women's Committees within the framework of the self-help organisations is imperative. Such committees can serve to work for the speical needs of women with disability. In addition, uneducated, rural and inexperienced disabled women are more likely to express themselves in a Women's Committee as the inhibitions imposed by socio-cultural patterns will not act as barriers to their participation.

Community-based rehabilitation services and out-reach programmes should be

established expeditiously. Such activities by the public and private sectors are the need of the day. Through these services women with disability can be reached and, along with the rendering of rehabilitiation services, can be trained to become contributing members of society.

Governments should involve women with disability in all activities that are concerned with the development of women in general. For this purpose, it is the responsibility of the self-help organisations to keep government departments aware of the role being played by women with disability in their own rather restricted fields.

The role of the United Nations, its agencies, NGOs working in the field of disability, development of women and providers of financial support, consultancy services and expertise has already been identified as an important means of development of leadership in women with disabilities. However, it should be emphasised once again that the widest distribution of these facilities should be made through co-ordinated efforts at all levels.[2]

Leadership training seminars have also been held especially for blind women in Kuala Lumpur, Malaysia (April 1981); Addis Ababa, Ethiopia (August 1982); Zambia (August 1982); Zimbabwe (December 1982); India (October 1983); São Paulo, Brazil (July 1985); and Islamabad, Pakistan (March 1986).

Self-confidence – which opens up new horizons for disabled women – is built on personal achievement. A young woman who is disabled moves into her own flat and organizes her abilities to live alone – she is out from under the over-protective family wing; a blind woman directs activities in an African open-air market – she

has come out of her housebound isolation; a thalidomide-injured young woman with short arms performs routine chores as a sailboat's crew member – she has found new ways to overcome her handicap.

While proving to herself that disability does not necessarily rule out personal achievement, the motivated disabled woman is also proving to a sceptical non-disabled world that its typical image of women with disability as dependent, objects of pity and charity, could not be further from the truth.

The three goals of the United Nations Decade for Women – equality, development and peace – are all equally important and inseparable in order to improve the condition of disabled women. And another important message of the decade is that it is only when women themselves fight that they can get closer to these goals. They need awareness, organisation, sisterhood and action. For this purpose, regional networks of handicapped women sharing experience and knowledge are invaluable.[3]

INTERVIEW WITH ROSANGELA BERMAN BIELER OF BRAZIL

The following is based on an interview with Rosangela Berman Bieler of Copacabana, Brazil, in May 1989 on the topic of women with disabilities. She was interviewed by Barbara Duncan, Assistant Secretary-General of Rehabilitation International. Rosangela is a leader of the disability advocacy movement in Brazil, where she has been responsible for producing *Etapa*, the newspaper of the movement, as well as organizing several regional and national seminars on disability policy and independent living. Currently she is employed by the Partners of the Americas to undertake information dissemination on the Partners New Technologies project as well as major

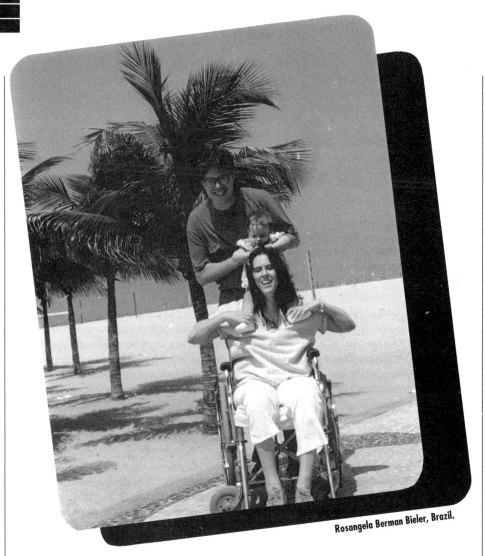

Rosangela Berman Bieler, Brazil.

developments in disability and rehabilitation.

Following negotiations with the government, and with the support of the office of the wife of the President of Brazil, Brazil's first independent living centre is now in the planning stages. Rosangela, together with a group of approximately ten other professionals, most of whom are disabled, will be in charge of developing and administering the centre. Rosangela has also been an active consultant with the mass media in Brazil, most recently assisting with the script and interpretation of a main character with a disability on a popular Brazilian soap opera. She uses a wheelchair.

Q: *Could you explain your philosophy about integrating disabled women's activities into overall disability advocacy projects?*

A: I personally feel that in Brazil we have so few leaders with disabilities that to focus on this issue in particular would spread us too thin. We find it much more important to give support to the participation of disabled men and women in all social movements and minority activities. For

86

example, in Brazil the Black minority groups, the gay groups, the women's movement have all been invited to take part in our leadership development seminars and we, on the other hand, actively support their movements. There are many popular organizations in Brazil, all of which have been charged with new energies following the dictatorship period, but we are all small and must work together to achieve any progress. We are too fragmentary to create a separate disabled women's movement and I think it would be better to merge disabled women with the few progressive organizations that exist. We know that the situation of disabled women and men can only advance when the general situation of the Brazilian people becomes better.

Q: *What have you experienced personally as a disabled woman that would differ from the experiences of a disabled man in the same situation?*

A: Well, I feel that my personal experiences have been lucky, that my life is lucky, but I also realize that this is often not the case with other disabled women. We have promoted many debates about sexuality, for example with some women and men who are disabled, and it is certainly evident that in Brazil and probably in all Latin American countries the culture will accept that disabled women must have 'good heads' but feel that their bodies can never express beauty. In other words, the aesthetic of our culture can permit men to have a certain bodily image and they can still date and get married because for women 'beauty is not the main thing in a relationship'. It's the same with persons with disabilities. Quite often, the disabled woman has lost her sexuality to her disability. She doesn't have the

right to use or to expose it in her life. I suspect that in all parts of the world this is largely the same and is due to cultural models of human beings and not due to a particular aspect of disability itself. This causes problems. We all know among us a disabled woman who has never had a kiss or a lover. This cultural process obviously interferes with equal opportunities in the job market, civil rights, etc.

My experience has been different in that my car accident was at age nineteen and I got married nine years after that. I met my husband Michael when I was disabled. But many people assume, and eventually let me know that they assume, that Michael was the person driving the car that caused my accident and married me because of guilt or some other reason like that. They cannot believe that an able-bodied man could fall in love with a disabled woman. People don't understand, either, how I became a mother who uses a wheelchair.

On this same topic, I recently saw a video tape (made by Bruce Curtis) of people in wheelchairs dancing. Even for me it was unusual to see an expression of beauty or art associated with a disabled body. I think there likely is this problem of associating beauty with disability for most of the public. I think it is up to disabled women, in a way, to become more attentive to this aspect of their lives. However, I think this particular approach should be dealt with within women's associations and groups which are already organized to deal with the demeaning status occupied by women in most countries.

My life is not so original; I just try to have a good balance right now between family, work and advocacy. I like myself as a woman, a disabled person and a human being. And it makes me happy and fulfilled. ●

IMAGINE A DOOR *

Karan McKibben, PhD

Over a decade ago, I first saw in my mind's eye the image of myself driving out of the front door in a motorized chair to a barrier-free university to pursue a graduate programme in English. What exactly was behind that front door and what exactly lay ahead at the university was quite vague, for the details of an independent life seemed more difficult to conceive than the determination to find more independence than I had found so far.

Now that I have earned a doctorate in English, am teaching composition at the University of California at Riverside, and living in my own condominium, I realize that the first image of the dream of independent living has been surpassed in many ways, while the goal behind that dream has undergone a more realistic redefinition. For me, an independent life has turned out to be an increasingly complex dependence on mechanical devices, people, and government programmes.

Since I contracted polio at the age of eight, I have been striving for as much independence as possible for a quadriplegic with respiratory involvement. This quest has led me to rely on an ever-changing and seemingly escalating array of equipment. Although too much equipment can be a disability in itself, each new advance in wheelchairs, ventilators, small buses, and various other devices has opened up new possibilities.

When I received my first motorized chair, at the age of thirteen, the concept of independence really dawned on me. This concept was given further impetus when-

ever my physical functioning was enhanced: by the rehabilitation work of Rancho Los Amigos Hospital, by the domestic arrangements of a home economist mother, by adaptive devices fashioned by a physicist father, and by such technological wonders as push-button telephones, remote-control televisions, electronic typewriters, and personal computers.

TECHNOLOGICAL BREAKTHROUGH

As new advances in respiratory equipment made it possible to replace the iron lung with increasingly more portable ventilators, travelling to family and professional affairs became easier. However, the advent of a small transport bus with a lift that could transport my motorized chair was the technological breakthrough that allowed me to think of myself finally as an independent person functioning in the world at large, not just in the home...

There was no college in my home town in New Mexico, and because my physical mobility was still rather limited, college began as one or two night classes but ended as an arduous affair of commuting to two different schools in nearby Santa Fe and Albuquerque, if 35 and 100 miles away can be called nearby. Nonetheless, eight years and over 20,000 miles later, I finally received a BA, a Phi Beta Kappa key, and $75 for being the top-ranked English major at the University of New Mexico. But this success in an undergraduate education did little to establish an independent lifestyle except to intensify a desire for it and to associate that desire with an equally intense one to attend graduate school...

After another year of commuting twice a week over the 100 miles to the University of New Mexico, it became clear that success in graduate school would

---

* *Rehabilitation Gazette*, Vol. 27, No. 2, 1986.

hardly be possible as long as I continued to live at home. Although we now had a small bus for transportation and I could use my motorized chair on campus, there were so many architectural barriers that I was still unable to participate fully and had to forgo the opportunities afforded by fellowships and teaching assistant-ships. Clearly, the proper equipment for maximum physical functioning and estab-lishing an academic reputation was not enough.

It was at this point that the image of the door to my own apartment and myself going off alone to a barrier-free university first began to crystallize. I soon realized that it could not happen in New Mexico because, at the time, the state did not pro-vide enough social services to enable a quadriplegic to live independently. The alternative of leaving home and moving to another state seemed not only intimidating but impossible to conceive. I had no answers to such vital questions as where to find a school without architectural barriers, how to pay for room and board, and where to obtain attendants and the money to pay for them. The New Mexico rehabilitation agency could only give me the advice that if I wished to achieve an independent life I would have to leave the state.

With much investigation, persistence, and luck, I finally found enough infor-mation to provide some realistic details to the fantasy image of my own front door. In California, there was a support system that would make an independent life-style possible for me. The University of California at Riverside (UCR) was one of the few universities that had made its campus totally accessible to disabled students and that had an extensive sup-port programme including wheelchair repair services, transportation in a small bus, library assistance, and attendant listings.

BUREAUCRATIC OBSTACLES

It was not easy to get governmental bureaucracies to communicate and co-operate. For example, New Mexico Division of Rehabilitation would pay for the first quarter of tuition but not at out-of-state rates, and California Division of Rehabilitation would pay for only the sec-ond quarter once I qualified for in-state fees.

Working out all the details proved to be a trying experience once I had actually moved nearly 1,000 miles away from my family and had begun to establish what I had imagined to be an independent lifestyle. After three moves within the first year, I found a small but workable two-bedroom apartment. When the apartment complex deteriorated, I located a more convenient condominium that my parents could invest in with the aid of my rent money.

After some misadventures with govern-mental bureaucracies, I learned how to get the support I needed and endure the inevitable hassles. After an illness or two, I found a medical support system I could rely on. After some near-disasters with attendant care, I learned how to depend on university students for personal care. After some frustrating moments with pub-lic transportation, the California Depart-ment of Rehabilitation helped me to obtain my own small bus. Although difficulties with individual links in this complex network of dependency on peo-ple, services, and mechanical devices threatened periodically to shatter my dream, finding solutions to these difficul-ties gradually improved my independent lifestyle and made its management easier, but never trouble-free.

Graduate school itself turned out to be easier to manage than maintaining myself independently, primarily because UCR's support for disabled students enabled me to concentrate on being simply a graduate student and not a physically handicapped student constantly battling against architectural barriers and physical limitation.

California's Department of Rehabilitation would not finance a PhD programme and a counsellor urged me to take an editing job. However, I decided to accept an assistantship because it promised to be more challenging and self-fulfilling, especially since I would be earning my tuition and some living expenses by teaching while studying. . . I finally received my degree in June 1985, well within the usual time for UCR's English programme. With this accomplishment it would seem my dream had been fulfilled. I not only have a PhD and a conveniently located condominium that I can call my own, but I also have a job teaching composition at UCR. Still, there is the realization that the independence I had first conceived is far from being realized. As a lecturer, I am still dependent on governmental support because I would have to teach too many classes to earn enough to replace that support. Although there is a good measure of satisfaction in teaching... I am looking for a more lucrative and fulfilling position so that I might lessen the network of support I currently depend on. It seems the life behind the door of my own original dream never ceases to unfold. The quest for independence has turned out to be a rather quixotic one that shapes an ongoing dream that can be realized only in the pursuit. ●

A SUCCESS STORY FROM NEPAL ☐ A brief case history of a blind girl in

Nepal, contributed by Amanda Hall, PhD, of the University of California, Berkeley, USA, shows that success stories of women with disabilities are not confined to those living in industrialized countries.

Twenty-eight-year-old Kamala K.C., who was born in a village 70 kilometres from Kathmandu, lost her sight as a result of an improperly treated eye infection she contracted at the age of two.

After studying at the Lab School in Kathmandu, an integrated school programme for blind children, Kamala was determined to continue her education. At the age of eighteen, she applied for entrance at the Mahendra Ratna College where she had to overcome the initial reluctance of college authorities to favour her application. She eventually convinced them that, despite her disability, she could do the required work. She not only completed her studies but went on to earn a Masters degree in history as well as doing graduate work in classical music.

Not content with academic achievement alone, Kamala has recently started her own school where she hopes to teach both disabled and non-disabled children.

1 Dr Fatima Shah, 'Issues concerning women with disability', Disabled People's International Asia–Pacific Leadership Training Seminar, Seoul, Republic of Korea, October 1986.
2 Dr Salma Maqbool, 'Development of leadership of women with disabilities', paper presented to the Leadership Training Seminar, Bangkok, Thailand, September 1988.
3 Yayori Matsui, 'UN Decade of Women and Special Concern of Disabled Women'.

ANNEX I
A GUIDE TO EDUCATION AND ACTION

> Action to help disabled women should not be left solely to the professionals. Any group, any organization, any individual can contribute.
>
> Specialists are not needed to pressure local authorities to ensure access for the disabled to public buildings, nor are they needed to raise public awareness and change negative attitudes that erode the self-confidence of disabled women and isolate them from the non-disabled world. Disabled women do not ask for much, just to be treated as human beings.

'WHATEVER IMPROVES THE STATUS of women generally will improve the status of disabled women' – a recurring conclusion of many groups and organisations – is basically true. But this maxim may easily be interpreted as meaning that disabled women, hoping for the best, simply wait passively for the progress won by their non-disabled sisters to trickle down and improve their own lives – and they may wait a long time or be by-passed entirely.

What relevance would a feminist victory winning equal pay for equal work have for an untrained, unemployed and perhaps over-protected woman who is disabled?

COMPLEMENTARY ACTION

While it is true that many organisations and agencies exist primarily to help the disabled, they are too often male-oriented and are still woefully inadequate in meeting the needs of millions of women. Action complementary to their services and to the various movements in favour of women is sorely needed.

Disability should be everyone's concern – not just that of rehabilitation professionals. Any organisation or programme for the general population can do something positive and practical, and the key word is 'practical'.

> Disabled women do not necessarily need specialized help – existing women's groups could make valuable contributions merely by expanding their areas of concern.

Widely varying degrees in the severity of disability, as well as vast differences in social and cultural backgrounds among women with disability, rule out hard-and-fast rules that would have universal application for aid to disabled women. And certainly, this book can present only a small part of the total picture and has no pretension to be a 'how-to' manual. Only women who have disabilities know and can point out the most challenging obstacles that stand between them and complete integration into the social and economic life of their societies.

Ruby Gonzales, living in the Philippines, is familiar with both the disabled and the non-disabled worlds – now using a wheelchair, she acquired her disability as a result of a car accident – and she takes a sober view of the shortcomings of some organisational efforts. She offers a clear outline of the special issues that generally reflect the primary concerns of women with disabilities and adds some suggestions for possible action.*

I note with great interest the recent flurry of activities worldwide that, in one way or another, deal with the women-and-disability issue particularly

---
* Excerpt from Ruby Gonzales, 'Employment: women with disabilities', Conference papers, n.d.

91

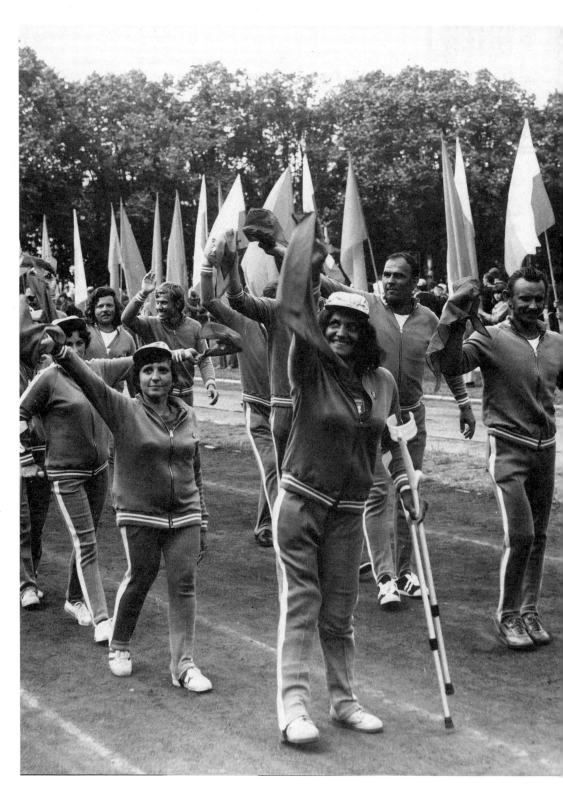

those that cover the Third World. A caucus on the problems of disabled women was held in Kenya; a Southern Africa regional workshop on vocational rehabilitation and employment of disabled women was held in Zimbabwe; and a women and disability project covering the Asia–Pacific region was undertaken, to name a few. We have recently concluded the UN Decade for Women. We are just beyond the middle of the Decade of Disabled Persons. We have a World Programme of Action Concerning Disabled Persons that specifically includes disabled women as a special group that deserves special attention.

Most of these have invariably resulted in the adoption of measures and policy recommendations that, altogether, are designed to give equal status to disabled women and to enable them to participate fully in community life. Sizeable though not complete statistics and data on the status problems and needs of disabled women have likewise been amassed.

Based on my experience, however, there is a great gap between the formulation of measures and policy recommendations and the actual implementation of concrete steps to improve the lot of disabled women which largely remains yet to be done. We generally know the problems and needs of our disabled women.. . . Concrete strategies based on the following suggestions for action could help meet those needs and solve at least some of the problems.

Proper attitudes of the public and of disabled women are essential. In the process of their integration into society, proper attitudes could develop into the public's wholehearted support and acceptance and into disabled women's [greater] confidence and determination to participate. Awareness campaigns, however, are necessary if attitudes concerning disabled women are to be changed. These information campaigns should address and tailor their messages to different audiences, namely: government, rehabilitation institutions, the general public and disabled women themselves.

A great majority of agencies, private and government, do not undertake special programmes and services for disabled women. Perhaps participatory planning workshops, involving these agencies, can be organised whereby awareness of

women-and-disability issues could be created as well as the adoption of steps to support them could be stimulated. Specifically, the representatives of the various agencies themselves will be asked to formulate plans and strategies to be implemented for the full integration and participation of disabled women in the community. Participation in the planning process may even lead to higher motivation.

If agencies continue to act on an individual basis, as they tend to do, already scarce resources would be further diffused. Much can be gained, therefore, if existing facilities and resources, programmes and services can be pooled and channelled to where they are urgently needed. A system of networks or formal linkages should be adopted. Information on facilities, programmes and services and resources offered could be exchanged. Through referrals to other agencies, an organisation could make a wider range of programmes and services available to disabled women.

Despite concentration of disabled women in rural areas most rehabilitation and disability-related agencies are urban-based and employ few, if any, field workers. Even the field personnel of the social welfare and health agencies are too few to bring help to enormous numbers of disabled in need. Furthermore, data suggest that within communities disabled women seem to know each other personally. It might be helpful to set up disabled women's organisations at village level. These groups could act as a receiver system for medical assistance, vocational/skills training and financial assistance for self-employment ventures, as conduits of information on job opportunities, as take-off points for business undertakings, as well as to assist the various agencies in their undertakings. It is further expected that the camaraderie and the discovery of potentials through group experiences will serve to instil pride and confidence among disabled women – so necessary if they are to be integrated into society without feelings of inferiority or self-pity.

Economics is central to alleviating the plight of disabled women. All avenues towards providing disabled women with gainful and fulfilling employment should be explored.

Many disabled women are not aware of agencies

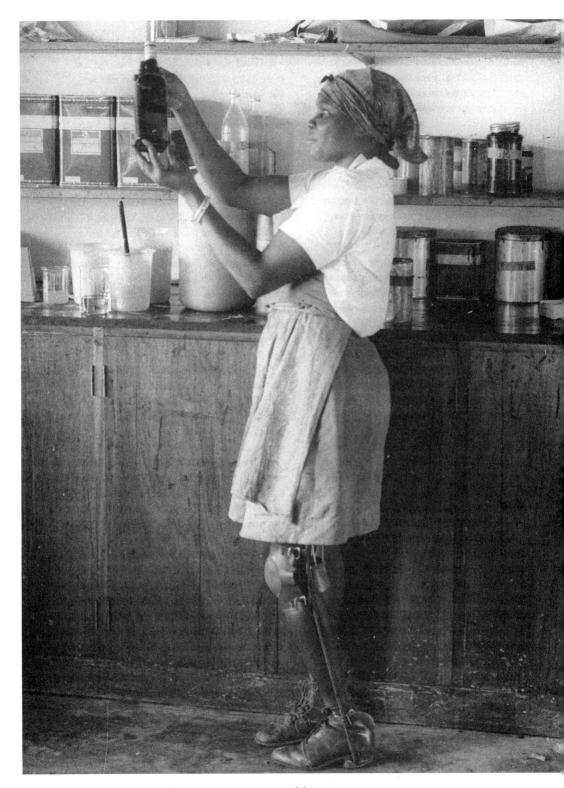

assisting the disabled. Furthermore, they are not aware of the service and programmes offered by these agencies. Medical information and news on available job opportunities are also needed. An information campaign concerning such topics as the existence of rehabilitation agencies and the range of services/programmes they offer, job opportunities available, and health advocacy ought to be carried out primarily by field workers by word of mouth. Due to the limited number of field personnel available, the campaign can be channelled through the proposed disabled women's organisations rather than to individuals. This can also be backed up through the use of media. In rural areas, radio and local comics and magazines could be appropriate channels.

Due mainly to financial limitations, very few disabled women can get medical services. Agencies, private and government, should collaborate to provide both medical advice on prevention and free or low-cost medical services preferably at the village levels to either cure or prevent the further deterioration of the disabled woman's condition. Representations should also be made to concerned organisations (for example, pharmaceutical companies, civic organisations, religious organisations, international aid bodies) to secure assistance in terms of personnel medicines and technical aids.

Finally, it is important to remember that there is no one-shot solution to the problems facing disabled women. Not even the most effective attitudinal and motivational campaign can succeed if disabled women continue to live in abject poverty, for example. Only combined and co-ordinated efforts can solve the problems facing disabled women today.

HOW GROUPS CAN PLAN FOR CHANGE

Existing women's groups, in addition to making special efforts to extend membership to women who have disabilities, could expand their areas of concern to include women with disability in their locality.

Specialised help is not always needed, for example, to increase opportunities, to improve access of disabled women to

assistance and to change negative attitudes. Much can be accomplished by the following:

● Encouraging the media and other institutions in the community to devote more attention to the situation of women with disabilities, helping them to do so by providing good speakers and good material, including articles by disabled women and interviews with them and their families.

● Encouraging the integration of disabled children in local schools and recreational activities by appropriate preparation of teachers, students and parents of both disabled and non-disabled children.

● Ensuring a follow-up to new community awareness by visiting restaurants, cinemas, theatres, public offices, schools and shops with physically handicapped people to determine whether they are accessible and, if not, keeping up pressure until they are.

● If necessary, supporting the right to education and training for all women and insisting that women who are disabled share this right.

● Arranging for educators, local employers and union representatives to meet disabled women and discuss employment problems and opportunities.

● Supporting the development of appropriate technology for work performed by women, with adaptation where necessary for disabled women.

● Starting community-based rehabilitation programmes.

● Encouraging development education, emphasising the relationships between poverty and disability, both locally and globally.

● Urging governments and non-governmental groups to accord higher

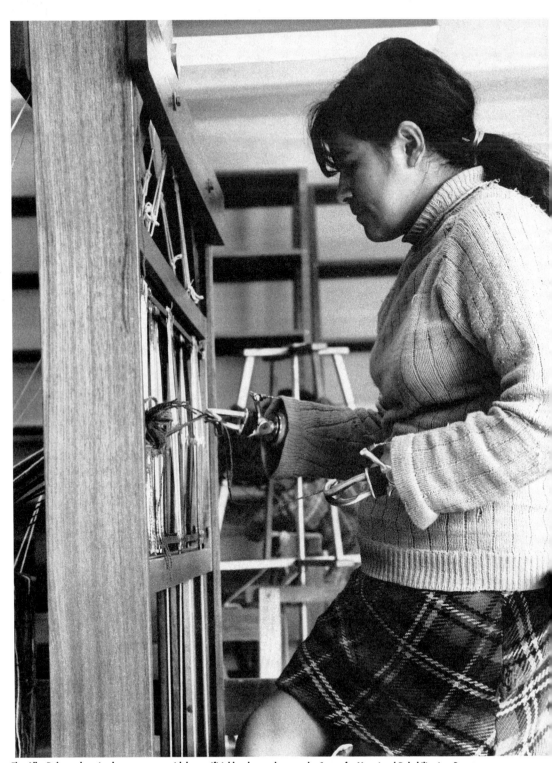

Flor Alba Roberto, learning how to weave with her artificial hands on a loom at the Centre for Vocational Rehabilitation, Bogota.

priority to programmes for primary health care, including immunisation, good nutrition, safe water and sanitation, and literacy.

FAMILIES NEED SUPPORT

Many groups could devote their efforts toward helping the families of women and girls who have disabilities. They, too, need support and services, which may include:

- Arranging contacts with other families coping with similar problems and encouraging self-support groups.
- Helping parents to develop positive attitudes that focus on the disabled family member's potential for normal development, not on her handicap.
- Compiling information about special services available for the disabled that would be useful to the families of women with disabilities.

Meetings, seminars and workshops are the tried-and-true means to a constructive end for most group action. They all have characteristics in common and may have different goals.

Generally speaking, *meetings* are held to discuss business, to make decisions and to plan follow-up action; they may be run according to strict rules or on an informal and flexible basis. *Seminars* are more ambitious and consist of several sessions over a period of several days for the purpose of discussing and exchanging ideas. They usually aim at producing a document, a work programme or recommendations. *Workshops* can be characterised as 'learning by sharing' experiences, which actively engage each participant and are usually carried out in conjunction with a seminar.

All three activities should have: a well-defined purpose, an agenda and timetable and a competent person in charge who can lead and guide discussions.

Meetings are, perhaps, the most flexible of these activities and may, for example, be merely informal get-togethers in a rural village of several women who are disabled and seeking mutual support, together with non-handicapped participants.

PLANNING A SEMINAR

Well-established organisations may find the material in this book useful as a basis, or at least a take-off point, to plan a seminar to spark off locally oriented action to help women with disability.

The Asian and Pacific Centre for Women and Development has drawn up a list of useful guidelines – reproduced below – for planning and conducting a seminar:

1. Be sure about the purpose of the seminar.

2. Organise speakers/experts well in advance to give them time to prepare for the seminar and prepare their papers on particular topics.

3. Arrange advance media coverage if you wish to have the purpose of the seminar made publicly known. Invite the media to cover the seminar if you want the message and outcome made known to a wider audience.

4. Select a skilled chairperson who can gauge when to adjourn or to break up into group discussions.

5. Identify resource people who can act as group discussion leaders and rapporteurs who will write down the main ideas. In the absence of skilled rapporteurs some advance training is recommended to ensure that group discussions are adequately reflected in the plenary session or in the final report.

6. Select participants according to the objectives of the seminar. Ask them to bring their experiences in written form, pictures or on tapes, for use in the workshop sessions.

7. Choose an environment appropriate to the seminar topic, for example, at the village level if related to the rural (disabled) poor.

8. Provide basic facilities and ensure adequate working space as well as secretarial and clerical support for participants.

9. Consider the use of audiovisual material – tapes, slides, charts – as tools to provide the focus for discussion.

10. Have a definite schedule prepared to present to participants and stress the goals to be achieved within that timescale.

11. As an introduction, arrange an informal session to allow participants to become acquainted. This will encourage a relaxed atmosphere and free exchange of views.

12. At the start of the seminar, make its purpose clear to the participants.

13. The organiser should have some idea of the anticipated outcome and be prepared to intervene and state this.

14. Do not overtax participants, particularly on the first day. Allow adequate time for private study and social activities.

15. To maintain interest and alertness, plan a range of approaches – practical exercises, simulated games, 'brainstorming', breaking into small groups, etc.

16. Ensure ongoing evaluation and feedback to participants.

17. Allow flexibility according to what evolves in the course of the seminar and do not rule out any alternatives.

18. Try to overcome cultural barriers through observation and sensitivity.

19. Follow up the seminar with analysis and evaluation.

The focus of seminars organised to discuss women-and-disability issues would depend, of course, on the preoccupations of the organising group.

The outline that follows, together with the guide-lines above, can assist in planning and holding a seminar. The outline is based on a five-day time frame and is for a group of not more than thirty-five participants, discussing predetermined topics.

It is suggested that morning sessions begin at 09:00 hours, a lunch hour be scheduled at 12:30 hours, with work resuming at about 14:00 hours and continuing to 17:00 hours. Coffee breaks during morning and afternoon sessions should be scheduled at convenient times. Evenings should – as far as possible – be work-free.

It is, however, advisable to organise a steering committee, meeting every evening to evaluate the day's activities and plan for the following day.

SUGGESTED OUTLINE FORMAT FOR SEMINAR

In the example overleaf, it is assumed that the purpose of running the seminar is (1) to inform people about the contents of this book and (2) to encourage creative thinking in order to come up with new and innovative kinds of activities.

This seminar is organised to promote maximum participation and discussion among participants. It is also arranged to encourage all participants to formulate their own ideas about what they personally can do to bring about change, upon returning to their own locality.

It is best, wherever possible, to use videos, films, photos, etc. in order to stimulate interest.

	FIRST DAY	SECOND DAY	THIRD DAY	FOURTH DAY	FIFTH DAY
MORNING	Registration of participants Self-introductions Why the meeting is being held and its objectives; how it will be run, etc. Assign participants to small working groups for the week	Review chapter 2 of book in plenary session Discuss related questions on chapter 2 in small work groups Summarise results of work groups in plenary session	Review chapters 3 and 4 in plenary session Discuss related questions on chapters 3 and 4 in small work groups Summarise results of work groups in plenary session	Review chapter 7 of book, in plenary session Discuss related questions on chapter 7 in small work groups Summarise results of work groups in plenary session	Ask each participant to put on paper what he/she can plan to bring about change or improvement Plenary session: discuss conclusions and recommendations for future
AFTERNOON	Review chapter 1 of book in plenary Discuss related questions on chapter 1 in small work groups Summarise results of work groups in plenary session	Invite disabled woman or group of women to talk on specific topic or arrange for visit to interesting local organisation	Review chapters 5 and 6 in plenary session Discuss related questions on chapters 5 and 6 in small work groups Summarise results of work groups in plenary session	Review annex 1 of book in plenary session Begin small group discussions on what concrete action can be taken (no plenary session)	Continue plenary discussion on conclusions and recommendations Final summation Closing ceremony

ANNEX II
LIST OF
ORGANISATIONS*

UNITED NATIONS SYSTEM

IMPACT (An International Initiative Against Avoidable Disability) c/o WHO, Room L. 225, 20 Avenue Appia, CH-1211 Geneva 10, Switzerland.

International Labour Organisation (ILO) Vocational Rehabilitation Branch, 4 route des Morillons, CH-1211 Geneva 22, Switzerland.

United Nations Centre for Social Development and Humanitarian Affairs Disabled Persons Unit, Vienna International Centre, PO Box 500, A-1400 Vienna, Austria.

United Nations Children's Fund (UNICEF) UNICEF HOUSE, 3 United Nations Plaza, New York, NY 10017, USA.

United Nations Educational, Scientific and Cultural Organisation (UNESCO) Special Programmes Section, Division of Structures, Contents, Methods and Techniques of Education, 7 place de Fontenoy, 75700 Paris, France.

United Nations High Commissioner for Refugees (UNHCR) 154 rue de Lausanne, CH-1211 Geneva 10, Switzerland.

World Health Organisation (WHO) Rehabilitation Section, 20 Avenue Appia, CH-1211 Geneva 10, Switzerland.

REGIONAL, INTER-GOVERNMENTAL ORGANIZATIONS

Bureau for Action in Favour of Disabled Persons Directorate General, Employment, Social Affairs and Education Commission of the European Community, rue de la Loi 200, B-1049 Brussels, Belgium.

Council of Europe Boite postale 431 R6 67006 Strasbourg Cedex France.

Organisation for Economic Co-Operation and Development* 2 rue André Pascal, 75775 Paris CEDEX 16, France.

Nordic Committee on Disability Fack, 161 25 Bromma, Sweden.

NON GOVERNMENTAL ORGANIZATIONS

AHRTAG Ltd. (Appropriate Health Resources and Technologies Action Group) 1 London Bridge St., London SE1.

Caribbean Association on Mental Retardation 6 Courtney Drive, Kingston 10, Jamaica.

Caritas Internationalis Piazza S. Calisto 16, 00153 Rome, Italy.

Disabled Women's Network (DAWN) c/o J. Meister, 776 E. Georgia Street, Vancouver, British Columbia, Canada V6A 2A3.

Equal Rights for Disabled Women Campaign 5 Netherhall Gardens, London NW3, UK.

European Alliance of Muscular Dystrophy Associations bd de Waterloo 115, 1000 Brussels, Belgium.

European Association for Special Education Secretariat, Box 79, Nordstrandhogda, 1112 Oslo 11, Norway.

Grupo Latinoamericano de Rehabilitación Profesional Apartado Aéreo 56208, Bogotá, DE, Colombia.

Handicap International 18 rue de Gerland, 69007 Lyon, France.

Helen Keller International Inc. 15 West 16th Street, New York, NY 10011, USA.

International Agency for the Prevention of Blindness c/o National Eye Institute, Building 31, Room 6A03, Bethesda, MD 20205, USA .

International Association of Parents of the Deaf 814 Thayer Avenue, Silver Springs, MD 20910, USA.

International Bureau for Epilepsy Achterweg 5, 2103, SW Heemstede, The Netherlands.

---

* This is a partial listing. For additional addresses and descriptions of programmes, see: ICOD Compendium: facts about the members of the International Council on Disability and related agencies of the United Nations system. Published by Rehabilitation International (address below, Non-Governmental Organisations)

International Cerebral Palsy Society 5a Netherhall Gardens, London NW3 5RN, UK.

International Committee of the Red Cross 17 rue de la Paix, CH-1211 Geneva, Switzerland.

International Council on Social Welfare Kostlergasse 1/29, A-1060 Vienna, Austria.

International Federation of Disabled Workers and Civilian Handicapped Reichsbund Auslandsreferat, Beethovenallee 56–58, 5300 Bonn 2, Germany.

International Federation of Physical Medicine and Rehabilitation c/o Medical College of Wisconsin, Curative Rehabilitation Center, 1000/N 92nd Street, Milwaukee, WI 53226, USA.

International League of Societies for Persons with Mental Handicap 248 Avenue Louise, 1050 Brussels, Belgium.

International Leprosy Association c/o Leprosy Mission, 5 Amrita Shergill Marg, New Delhi 110 003, India.

International Society for Prosthetics and Orthotics Borgervaenget 5, 2100 Copenhagen 0, Denmark.

League of Red Cross and Red Crescent Societies PO Box 276, CH-1211 Geneva 19, Switzerland.

Physically Handicapped and Able-Bodied Tavistock House North, Tavistock Square, London WC1H 9HJ, UK.

Rehabilitation International 25 East 21st Street, New York, NY 10010, USA.

Royal Commonwealth Society for the Blind Commonwealth House, Heath Road, Haywards Heath, West Sussex RH16 3AZ, UK.

Soroptimist International of the Americas 1616 Walnut Street, Philadelphia, PA 19103, USA.

World Association for Psychosocial Rehabilitation PO Box 898 Ansonia Station, New York, NY 10023, USA.

World Blind Union 58 avenue Bosquet, 75007 Paris, France.

World Confederation for Physical Therapy 16–19 Eastcastle Street, London W1N 7PA, UK.

World Federation of Occupational Therapists 2375 Cote Ste.-Catherine, Montreal H3AT 1A8, Canada.

World Federation of the Deaf 120 Via Gregorio VII, 00165 Rome, Italy.

World Institute on Disability 1720 Oregon Street, Suite 4, Berkeley, CA 94703, USA.

ANNEX III

ADDITIONAL READING*

GENERAL

Awake: Asian women and the struggle for justice. Published by Asia Partnership for Human Development, 154 Elizabeth Street, Sydney, NSW 2000, Australia, 1985. 127 pp.

Disability Studies Quarterly (a magazine that covers issues on women and disability). Published by Brandeis University, Department of Psychology, Waltham, MA 02254, USA.

Disabled Women and Development Issues: some observations. By Susan Sygall, Mobility International USA, PO Box 3551, Eugene, OR 97403, USA.

Disabled Women in America: a statistical report drawn from Census Bureau data. The President's Committee on Employment of the Handicapped, Washington, DC 20210, 1984. 26 pp.

Disabled Women's Issues (discussion paper). By April D'Aubin, published by Coalition of Provincial Organizations of the Handicapped, 926–924 Portage Avenue, Winnipeg, Manitoba, K3C 089, Canada.

Dispelling the Shadows of Neglect: a survey on women with disabilities in six Asian and Pacific Countries. ILO, Geneva, 1989. 29 pp.

Eminent Blind Women of the World: their contribution and achievements. By Usha Bhalerao, published by Sterling Publishers Private Ltd., L-10 Green Park Extension, New Delhi 110016, 1988. 118 pp.

Empowering Women Workers: the WWF experiment in Indian cities. Published by Working Women's Forum (WWF), 55 Bheemasena Garden Road, Mylapore, Madras 600–004, India, 1986. 182 pp.

International Rehabilitation Review. Published three times yearly by Rehabilitation International, 25 East 21st Street, New York, NY 10010, USA, annual subscription US$30.

Leadership Training Seminar, Report of DPI Asia–Pacific (with focus on disabled women). Published by Asia/Pacific Regional Council of DPI, Sangiin-Kaikan 210, 2-1-1 Nagata-cho, Chiyoda-ku, Tokyo 170, 1986. 152 pp.

Nairobi Forward-Looking Strategies for the Advancement of Women. United Nations, Nairobi, 1986. 89 pp.

Proceedings of the 16th World Congress of Rehabilitation International, Tokyo. Published by the Japanese Society of Rehabilitation of the Disabled, 1-22-1 Toyama, Shin–juku, Tokyo, 162, 1989.

Tribune: women and development quarterly bulletin. Published by the International Women's Tribune Center, 777 UN Plaza, New York, NY 10017, USA.

Voices from the Shadows: women with disabilities speak out. By Gwyneth Ferguson Matthews, published by Women's Educational Press, Toronto, Canada, 1983.

Vox Nostra. Published by Disabled Peoples' International, DPI Headquarters, 504–352 Donald Street, Winnipeg, Manitoba, Canada, annual subscription US$15.

With the Power of Each Breath: a disabled women's anthology. Edited by Susan E. Browne, Debra Connors and Nanci Stern, published by Cleis Press, PO Box 8933, Pittsburgh, PA 15221, USA, 1985. 354 pp.

Women and Disability. Special issue of *Pro Infirmis*, Vol. 3, 1988, Redaktion Pro Infirmis, Feideggstrasse 71, Postfach 129, Zurich, 8032 Switzerland (in French, German, Italian).

Women and Disability: an issue. Produced by Women with Disabilities Feminist Collective, c/o COSGH, 247 Flinders Lane, Melbourne 3000, Australia. 75 pp.

Women and Girls with Disabilities: an introductory teaching packet. By Elizabeth

---

* Includes audio-visual documents

Phillips. Organisation for the Equal Education of the Sexes, Inc., 438 4th Street, Brooklyn, New York, NY 11215, USA, 1986.

'Women with disability' (paper presented at a Regional Expert Seminar to review achievements at the mid-point of the UN Decade of Disabled Persons), prepared by Dr Fatima Shah, 1987. Available from: DPI HQ, Box 360 33, S-100 71, Stockholm, Sweden. 12 pp.

IMAGES (SELF AND PUBLIC); SEXUALITY

Able Lives: women's experience of paralysis. Edited by Jenny Morris, published by The Women's Press, 34 Great Sutton Street, London EC1V 0DX, UK, 1989. 227 pp. £5.95.

The Body's Memory (a novel). By Jean Stewart, published by St Martin's Press, 175 Fifth Avenue, New York, NY 10010, USA.

Choices: a guide to sex counseling with physically disabled adults. By Maureen Neistadt and Maureen Freda, Robert Krieger Publishing Co., Malabar, Florida, USA, 1987.

Developing Strategies for Communications about Disability: experiences in the US, Hong Kong, India and Pakistan. By Barbara Kolucki, World Rehabilitation Fund, Inc., 400 East 34th Street, New York, USA, 1989.

Disabled, Female and Proud! By Marilyn Rousso, Exceptional Parent Press, Boston, 1988.

Discrimination Against Women: a global survey of the economic, educational, social and political status of women. By Eschel M. Rhoodie, published by McFarland and Co., Jefferson, North Carolina, USA, and London.

Positive Images: portraits of women with disabilities (VHS video). Published by Women Make Movies, 225 Lafayette Street, Suite 211, New York, NY 10012, USA.

Women's Health, Our Minds, Our Bodies.

Edited by Kathleen E. Grady and Jeanne Parr LemKau, special issue of *Psychology of Women Quarterly*, Vol. 12, No. 4, Cambridge University Press, 1988.

PREVENTION

Childhood Disability, Prevention and Rehabilitation. UNICEF Programme Guidelines, Vol. 8, 1987.

Measuring Reproductive Morbidity. Report of a Technical Working Group. WHO, Geneva, 30 August–1 September 1989.

Overview of the Health of Women and Children. WHO Technical Background Paper on Better Health for Women and Children Through Family Planning, Nairobi, 5–9 October 1987.

Prevention and Treatment of Obstetric Fistulae. Report of Technical Working Group. WHO, Geneva, 17–21 April 1989.

Study on Traditional Practices Affecting the Health of Women and Children. Preliminary report by Mrs H.E. Warzazi for United Nations Commission on Human Rights, Sub-Commission on Prevention of Discrimination and Protection of Minorities (E/CN.4/Sub.2/1989/42), August 1989 (in English, French, Spanish).

Women and Health, special issue of *World Health Statistics Quarterly*, Vol. 40, No. 3. WHO, 1987 (English/French).

WOMEN CARE-GIVERS

Tristan: physically and mentally handicapped ... socially and spiritually gifted. By Suzanne Schuurman, published by George Ronald, Oxford, 1987. 230 pp.

SELF-HELP, COMMUNITY-BASED REHABILITATION, AND SOCIAL INTEGRATION

Able Lives: women's experiences of paralysis. Edited by Jenny Morris, The Women's Press, 1989. 227 pp.

Building Community: a manual exploring issues of women and disability. Written by members of Women and Disability

Awareness Project. Published by Educational Equity Concepts Inc., 440 Park Avenue South, New York, NY 10016, 1985.

Disabled Village Children: a guide for community health workers, rehabilitation workers and families. By David Werner, published by Hesperian Foundation, PO Box 1692, Palo Alto, CA 94302, USA. 654 pp.

Experience and Reflections on a New Concept of Service Provision for Disabled People. By Willi Momm, Andreas König, ILO, Geneva, 1989.

First Year Report, 1988, of the Project on Women and Disability. 1 Ashburton Place, Room 1305, Boston, MA, 02108, USA.

I Always Wanted to be a Tapdancer - Women with Disabilities. Edited by Annee Lawrence. Available from: Women's Co-ordination Unit, Level 3, 31–39 Macquarie Street, Parramatta, 2150 Australia. 1989, 211 pp.

Manual – Training in Community for People with Disabilities (training pack for a family member of a person with disability). WHO, Geneva, 1988.

Organising a Meeting (DPI manual for national, regional and international meetings). DPI, 504–352 Donald Street, Winnipeg, Manitoba, R3B 2H8, Canada.

Women and Disability: an issue. Published by Women with Disabilities Feminist Collective and available from: WDFC, c/o COSHG, 247 Flinders Lane, Melbourne, 3000 Australia. 1988, 75 pp.

Women with Disabilities: essays in psychology, culture and politics. Edited by Michelle Fine and Adrienne Asch, published by Temple University Press, Philadelphia, PA, 19122, USA. 1988.

VOCATIONAL TRAINING AND EMPLOYMENT

Development of Policies and Programmes for Disabled Women and Female Disabled Children in the Southern African Region. Report of the workshop held in Harare, Zimbabwe. ILO, 1985.

Development of Policies and Programmes for Social and Vocational Rehabilitation for Disabled Women in the Middle East Region. Report of the Workshop held in Amman, Jordan. ILO, 1987, 79 pp. (also available in Arabic).

Integrating Disabled Women and Girls in Development and Income-Generating Projects. Report of the National Workshop held in Mbabane, Swaziland. ILO, 1987.

Socio-Vocational Integration of Disabled Women in Japan, an Analytic Report. By Dr Yoko Kojima, published by the Office of Social Rehabilitation Research, Villa Royal, Sanbancho 502, 7–2 Sanbancho, Chiyoda-ku, Tokyo, 102, 1988. 153 pp.

Standards and Policy Statements of Special Interest to Women Workers. ILO, Geneva, 1980. 132 pp.

Training Manual on the Transfer of Technology Among Rural Women, United Nations Economic and Social Commission for Asia and Pacific (ESCAP), Bangkok, 1987.

Vocational Rehabilitation of Disabled Women in the European Community. By Mary Croxen John for the Commission of the European Community's Bureau Actions in Favour of Disabled People, 1988.

Vocational Rehabilitation of Women with Disabilities. By Sheila Stace, ILO, Geneva, 1986. 38 pp., 12.50 Swiss francs.

Women with Disabilities: essays in psychology, culture and politics. Edited by Michelle Fine and Adrienne Asch, published by Temple University Press, 1988.

OLDER WOMEN AND AGEING

Network News (newsletter of the Global Link for Midlife and Older Women). Sponsored by the International Federation on Ageing, 449 Swanston Street, Melbourne, Victoria 300, Australia; supported by Women's Initiative of AARP, 1909 K Street, NW Washington, DC 20049, USA.

Women's Age Page Collection: health and personal care guidelines for ageing women. National Institute of Ageing, Information

Center/Women's AP, 2209 Distribution
Circle, Silver Spring, MD 20910, USA.

For a wide selection of publications on
women's issues in general:

Zed Books Ltd
57 Caledonian Road
London N1 9BU
UK

Zed Books Ltd
171 First Avenue
Atlantic Highlands
New Jersey 07716
USA

INDEX

ability, focus on, viii
acceptance, phase of, 10
accessibility, 16, 32, 55, 82, 91, 95
activity, phase of, 10
Afghanistan, 4
ageing, 73-78; and women, xi; and women
     carers, 76; changes associated with, 77;
     training programmes in, 77
ageism, 73, 75
aggression, phase of, 8-10
Angola, 4
appliances, local production of, 25
architectural barriers to disabled people, 89
arthritis, 74, 76
Asia and Pacific Centre for Women and
     Development, 97
athetosis, 36-8
Atlantic Ocean, crossing of, 81
Australia, x
awareness of public, of disability, 84, 95

Bangladesh, 4, 11-12, 29
Bhutan, 21
Bieler, Rosangela Berman, 85-8
biomedical developments, 1
birth attendants, traditional, 24
birth, injuries at, 3, 22
births, difficult, dangers of, 1
blind girls, pregnancy of, 46
blind people, 29; schools for, 13
blind women, 3-4, 43-8, 90; as dressmakers,
     29; as factory hands, 29; as market
     women, 48; as teachers, 29; training of,
     85
blindness, 12-13, 21; of children, 18
Bolivia, 21
Botswana, 25, 29
Braille, 77
Braille speech printers, 39
brain/computer interface, 39
Braun, Roswita, 6
Brazil, 85-8

cancer, 74
careers, non-traditional, 43; disabled
     women in, t45, t44

carers, xi, 12, 64-72; family as, 25; free
     choice of, 69; needs of, 66; women as, 6,
     64, 66-7, 69-72; women, and old age, 76
cerebral palsy, 70
certainty, phase of, 8
Chanel, Coco, 73
childbirth, and disabled women, 18, 61-2
childcare, 1, 46, 48; and disabled mothers,
     57
children: adaptation to parent's disability,
     62; blind, 18, 46; needs of, 41; right to
     bear, 55-7 see also disabled children
China, disabled children in, 34
churches, 7; attitudes to disabled people,
     15-17
circumcision, female, 19, 23
co-operative movement, of blind women,
     46-7
Coalition of Provincial Organisations of the
     Handicapped (Canada), 54
community care, 67
Community Welfare Promotion
     Foundation (Tokyo), 65
community-based care for elderly, 75
community-based rehabilitation, 25, 27;
     criticism of, 27
computer-based production processes, 38
computerised axial tomography, 36
computers, 39
Cornell University Medical College, 75
cottage industries, disabled women
     employed in, 31-2
crisis management, 7; phases of, 8-11
Curtis, Bruce, 87
custody of children, for disabled women, 55

dance: and blind women, 46; in
     wheelchairs, 87
data on disabled women: lack of, 41; need
     for, 19-21
day centres, for handicapped children, 71
de la Vega, Amelita, 79-80
death, 6; wish for, 8
depression, 12, 74; phase of, 10
deskilling as result of technological
     advance, 41
devil, as source of disability, 16
diabetes, 74